# Dr. Davenport's Insanely Easy Acid Reflux Cookbook

Tracy Davenport, Ph.D.

Copyright © 2018 Author Name
All rights reserved.
ISBN-13: 9781099356636

*For my mom…for all her kindness and support*

# Introduction

If you or someone in your family was just diagnosed with acid reflux disease or GERD, you probably already know that changing your diet is what you are supposed to try first. The National Institutes of Health and American College of Gastroenterology recommend that you reduce your intake of total fat, chocolate, alcohol, citrus, tomato products, coffee, and tea. However, we both know this can be harder than it sounds, especially if you are living a real life like I was when my son was born with severe acid reflux.

What you will find as you look ahead are recipes that are insanely easy enough that you can make them on just a little sleep, a small budget, and have the confidence that everyone in your family will find them delicious and healthy. Many of the recipes are gluten free and dairy free as gluten and dairy made my son's reflux worse. These are the recipes that were part of my survival guide while I tried to work, be a parent to both of my children, and save just a little bit of my sanity.

As you will soon find out, everyone's acid reflux is different, which means different people living with acid reflux tolerate different foods. So, if you find a recipe that looks good, but you know that it might require a slight modification for or your loved one, by all means just make the change. The recipes ahead are meant to save you time and help you get started on your journey.

As my kids say: LET'S GOOOOO!

## TABLE OF CONTENTS

| | |
|---|---|
| **Introduction** | **3** |
| **Chapter One: Breakfast** | **7** |
|     Apple French Toast Bake | 9 |
|     Carrot Cake Pancakes | 11 |
|     Coconut Apple Muffins | 13 |
|     Oatmeal Breakfast Bars | 15 |
|     Creamy Mango Smoothie | 17 |
|     Banana Split Smoothie | 19 |
| **Chapter Two: Snacks and Sides** | **21** |
|     Country Biscuits | 23 |
|     Grilled Plantains with Brown Sugar Glaze | 25 |
|     Potato-Zucchini Latkes | 27 |
|     Banana Bars | 29 |
|     Candied Bacon Sticks | 31 |
|     Cheese Crispas with Avocado | 33 |
| **Chapter Three: Sandwiches** | **35** |
|     California Burger | 37 |
|     Turkey Meatball Sub | 39 |
|     Tuna Salad Lettuce Wrap | 41 |
|     Almond Butter, Banana and Honey Sandwich | 43 |
|     Grilled Turkey Reuben | 45 |
|     Chicken Parmesan Sub | 47 |
| **Chapter Four: Entrees** | **49** |
|     Beef Stroganoff | 51 |
|     Shrimp Poke Bowls | 53 |
|     Chicken Spaghetti | 55 |

| | |
|---|---|
| Pork Chops with Gravy | 57 |
| Creamy Potato Soup | 59 |
| Shrimp Lo Mein | 61 |
| **Chapter Five: Desserts** | **63** |
| Autumn's Apple Cake | 65 |
| Cool Rice Pudding | 67 |
| Pina Colada Cookies | 69 |
| Walnut Dainties | 71 |
| Coconut Banana Freeze | 73 |
| Jam-Packed Lemon Cake | 75 |
| **From Tracy** | **77** |

# Chapter One: Breakfast

Breakfast can be a very difficult meal for many suffering from acid reflux. If you feel like your acid reflux symptoms are actually worst first thing in the morning, you are not alone. There is even a name for what you may be experiencing. It's called "riser's reflux." When my youngest son with reflux was young, my older son made him a breakfast menu of things that might make him feel better in the morning. Many mornings that he didn't feel well, he chose from that menu.

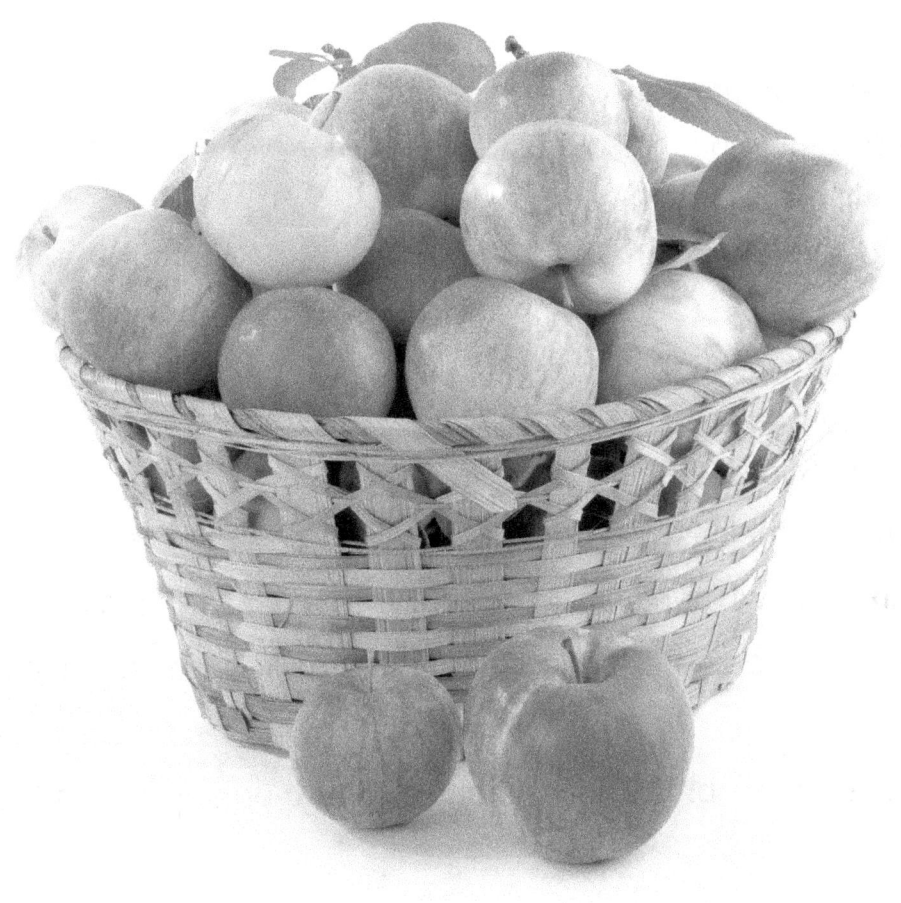

# Apple French Toast Bake

Serves 2

This breakfast dish is warm and filling but is still very easy on the stomach.

**Ingredients:**

Cooking spray
2 eggs, beaten slightly
pinch of salt
1 apple, peeled and cut into very small pieces
4 slices rice bread, cut into small cubes
1 splash of rice milk
4 Tbs. of maple syrup

**Directions:**

1. Preheat oven to 350 degrees.
2. Spray two small ramekins with cooking spray.
3. In a small mixing bowl, gently mix together the eggs, salt, apple, bread and milk.
4. When the bread is coated with the egg and the milk, pour the mixture into the ramekin.
5. Bake until the egg and bread set and begin to turn golden brown (about 10 – 15 minutes).
6. Remove from the oven and top with the maple syrup. Serve warm.

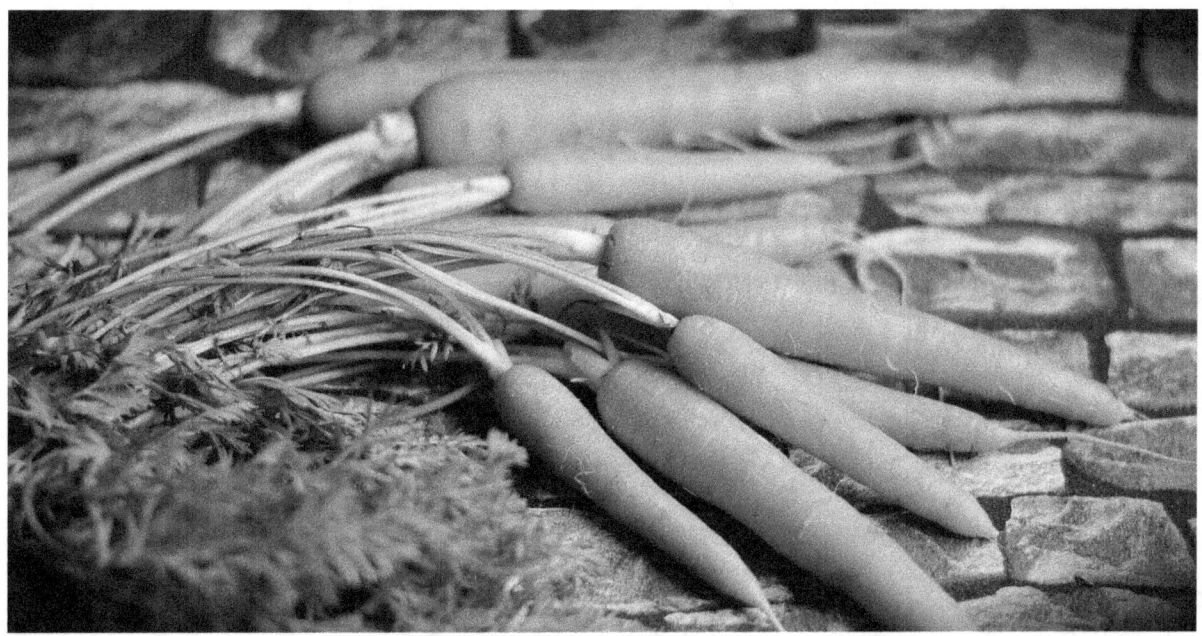

# Carrot Cake Pancakes

Serves 2-3

These pancakes are fun to eat and are light enough to be easy-on-the-stomach year-round.

**Ingredients:**

2 cups pancake mix (gluten free mix works well)
2 eggs
1 cup milk or milk substitute
2 Tbs. vegetable oil
½ cup shredded carrots
½ cup unsweetened crushed pineapple, drained
¼ cup chopped walnuts

¼ tsp. ground ginger

**Directions:**

1. Heat griddle to medium heat.
2. Place the mix in a bowl. Add the eggs, milk and oil and mix until thoroughly blended. Gently fold in the carrots, pineapple, walnuts and ginger.
3. Coat the griddle with non-stick cooking spray.
4. Ladle the pancakes onto the griddle.
5. Cook until pancakes bubble and then flip the pancakes to cook on the other side.
6. Remove from heat when they are golden brown on both sides.
7. Sprinkle lightly with powdered sugar before serving.

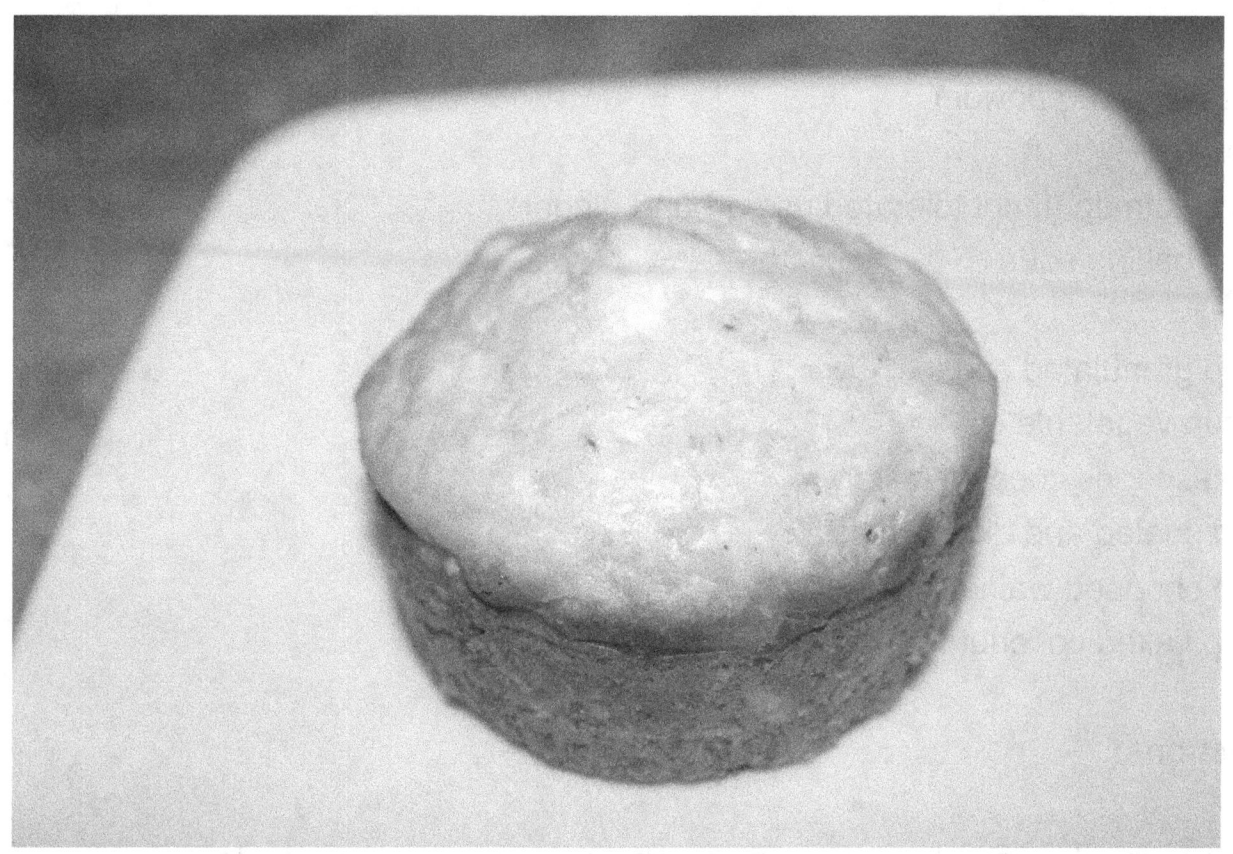

# Coconut Apple Muffins

Serves 4

These muffins are moist and chewy and make a great breakfast. They are also gluten free and dairy free.

**Ingredients:**

1 ½ cups oat flour
1 ½ tsp. baking powder
¾ tsp. salt
½ tsp. nutmeg (if not tolerated use ground ginger)
¼ tsp. baking soda
2 eggs
¾ cup granulated sugar
1/3 cup vegetable oil
3 tablespoons coconut milk
1 cup peeled and diced apples
1 cup chopped walnuts
¾ cup flaked coconut

**Directions:**

1. Combine the flour, baking powder, salt, nutmeg and baking soda.
2. In another bowl, beat eggs, sugar, oil and milk. Stir in the apples, nuts and coconut.
3. Stir the wet ingredients into the dry ingredients just until moistened.
4. Fill muffin cups 3/4 full.
5. Bake at 350 degrees for 20 – 25 minutes or until a toothpick comes out clean.

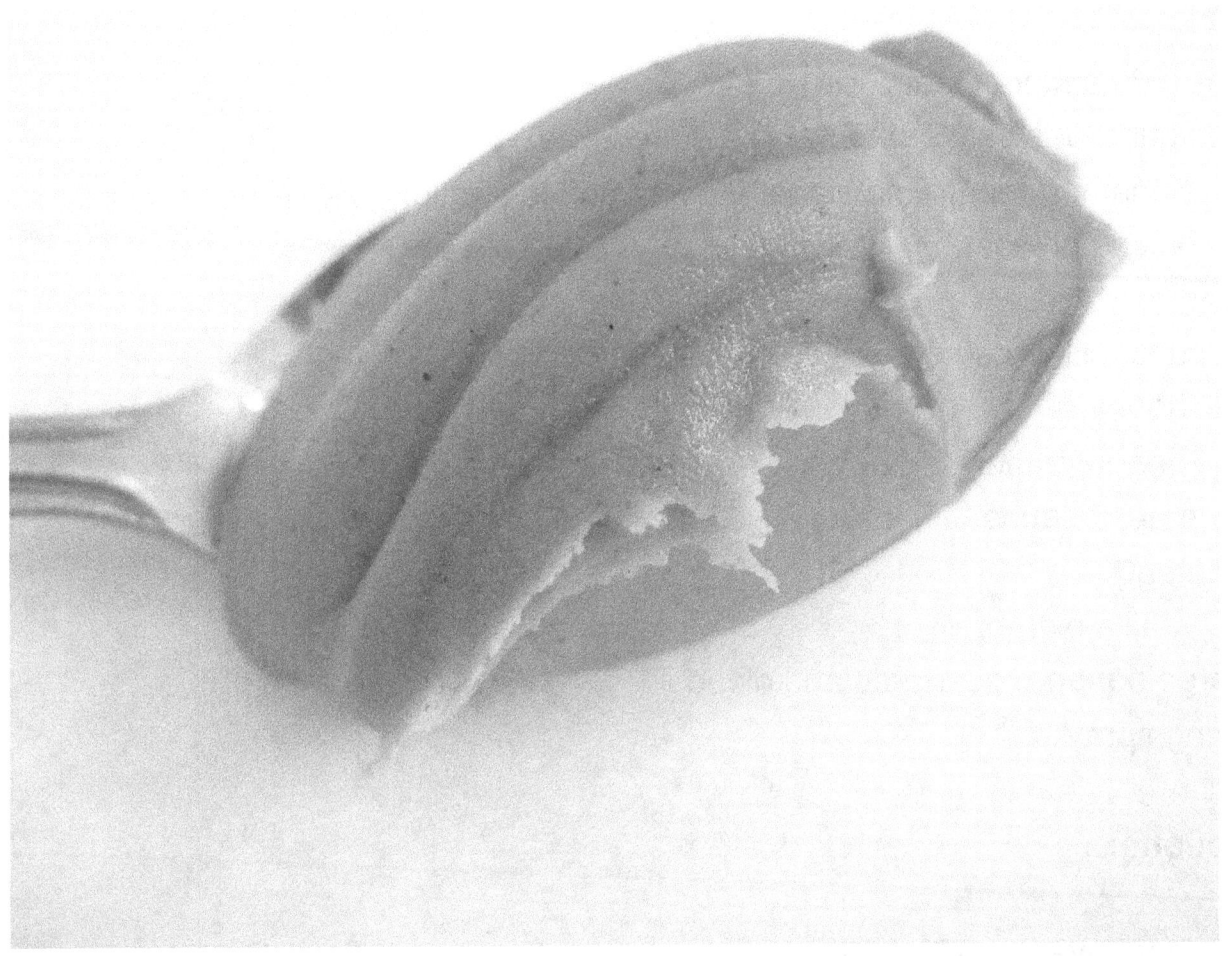

## Oatmeal Breakfast Bars

Makes an 8"x 8" pan

These bars are great when you need to eat breakfast on the run. I always made these bars to send with my oldest son back to college. They are super healthy and full of protein.

**Ingredients:**

2 cups old fashioned oats
1 cup flour (I use oat flour to make it gluten free)
2 tsp. cinnamon (or ground ginger if cinnamon is a reflux trigger for you)
1 tsp. baking powder
1/4 tsp. salt
1 1/2 cups milk (I use rice milk)
3 Tbs. honey
2 Tbs. peanut butter
1/2 cup applesauce
1 large egg
1 tsp. vanilla extract
1/2 large banana, quartered and diced
Cooking spray

**Directions:**

1. Preheat oven to 375 degrees.
2. Lightly coat an 8" x 8" pan with cooking spray.
3. In a medium bowl, combine the dry ingredients except for the banana.
4. In another bowl, stir together the milk, applesauce, egg, honey, peanut butter, and vanilla.
5. Pour the dry ingredients into the wet ingredients. Stir to combine. Fold the banana in.
6. Pour the batter into the pan and press to the sides. Bake for 35 minutes or until golden brown and a toothpick in the center comes out clean. Cool and cut into bars.

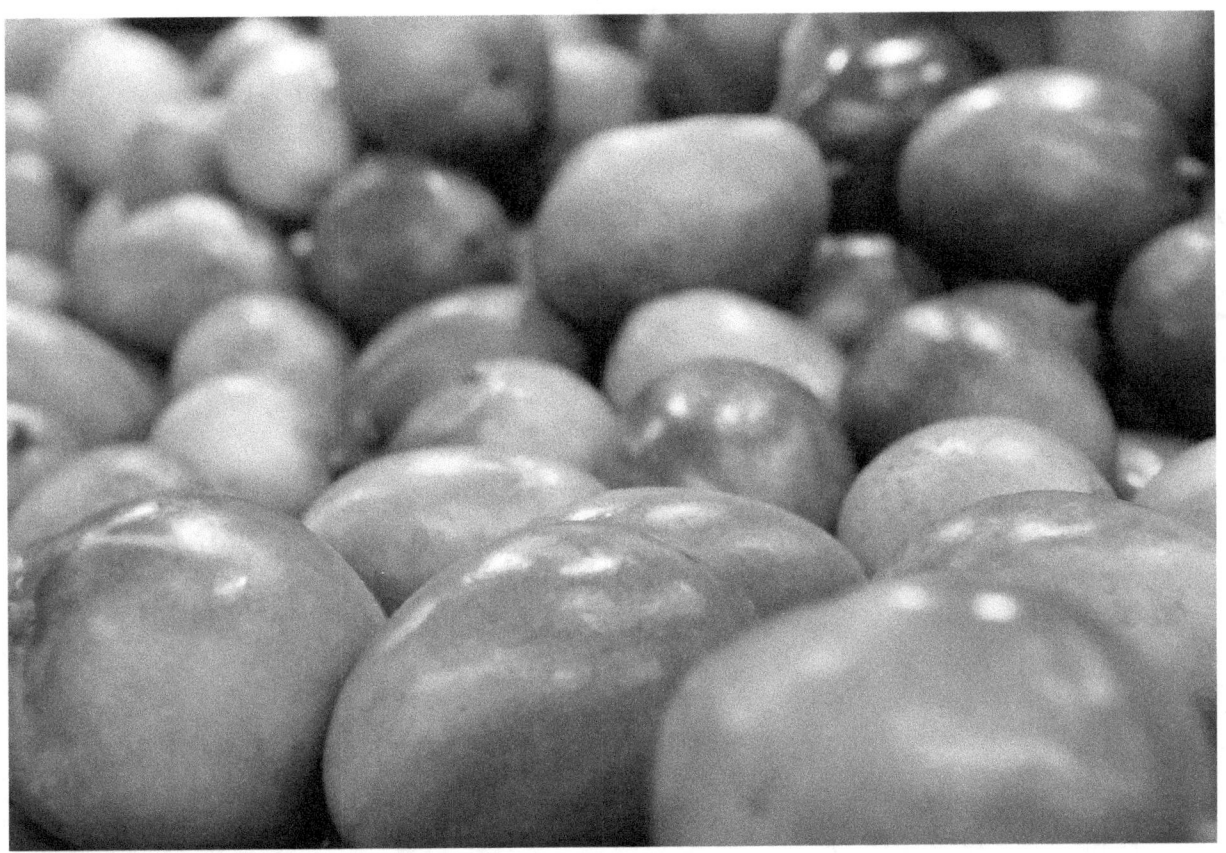

# Creamy Mango Smoothie

Serves 1

Smoothies are a great way to give your body the nutrients it needs while you are on the go. Mango is high in vitamin C and fiber and tastes great.

**Ingredients:**

1 cup coconut milk
1 dash vanilla extract
1/2 cup frozen mango

1/2 frozen and peeled banana

**Directions:**

1. Put coconut milk in the blender first.
2. Add the frozen fruit.
3. Mix until blended and smooth.
4. Serve.

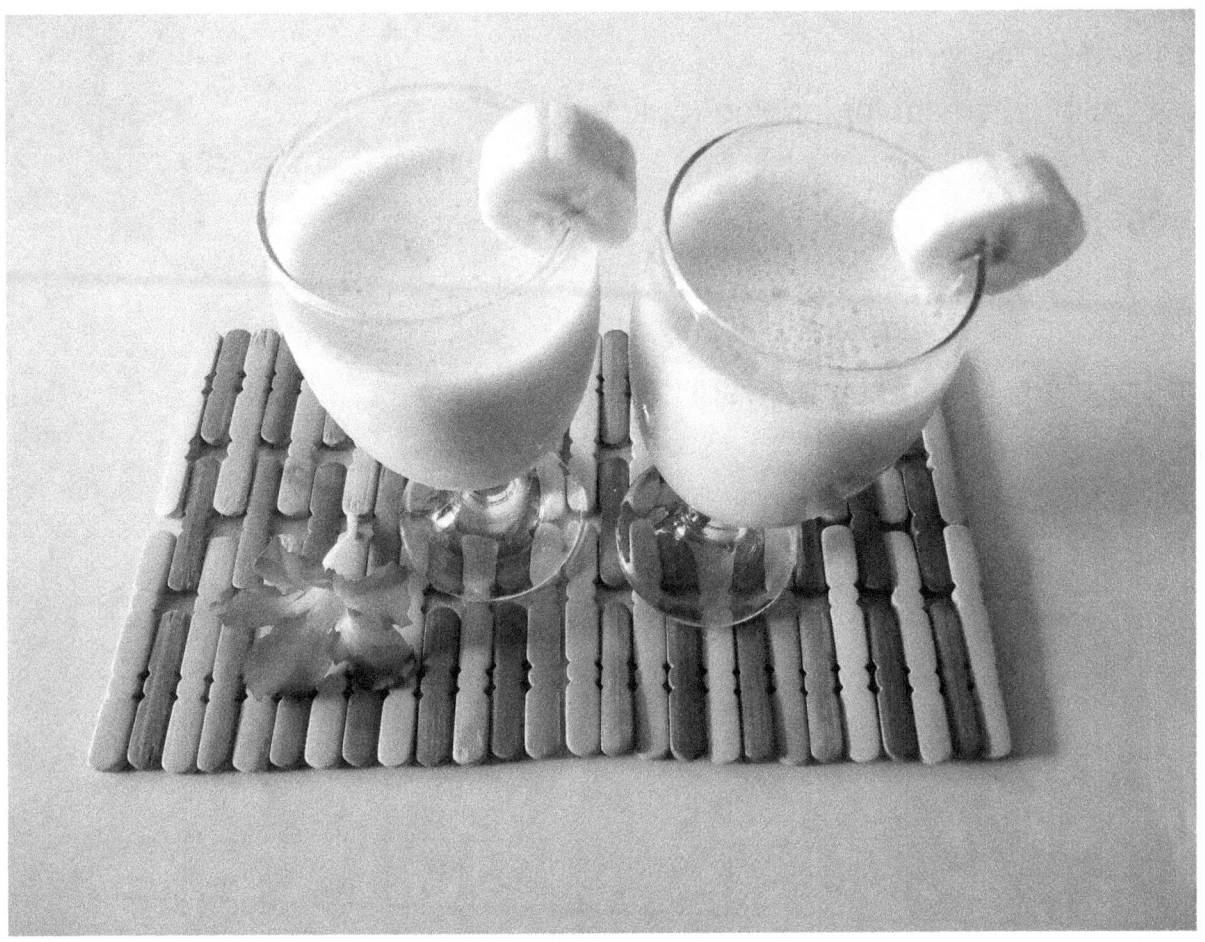

## Banana Split Smoothie

Serves 2

For those in your house with a sweet tooth, this smoothie is sure to satisfy.

**Ingredients:**

1 cup almond milk
2 medium bananas (ripe, peeled, and frozen)
1 Tbs. almond butter

½ tsp. vanilla extract
2 pitted dates
1 Tbs. shredded coconut
Coconut whipped cream for topping (optional)

**Directions:**

1. Add almond milk to the blender.
2. Add bananas, almond butter, vanilla, and dates.
3. Blend until smooth.
4. Top with whipped cream and coconut before serving.

# Chapter Two: Snacks and Sides

Snacks and side dishes are often high in fat and sugar. The secret is to make them as fun as possible, but without the high fat, high sugar content that often accompanies snacks and side dishes.

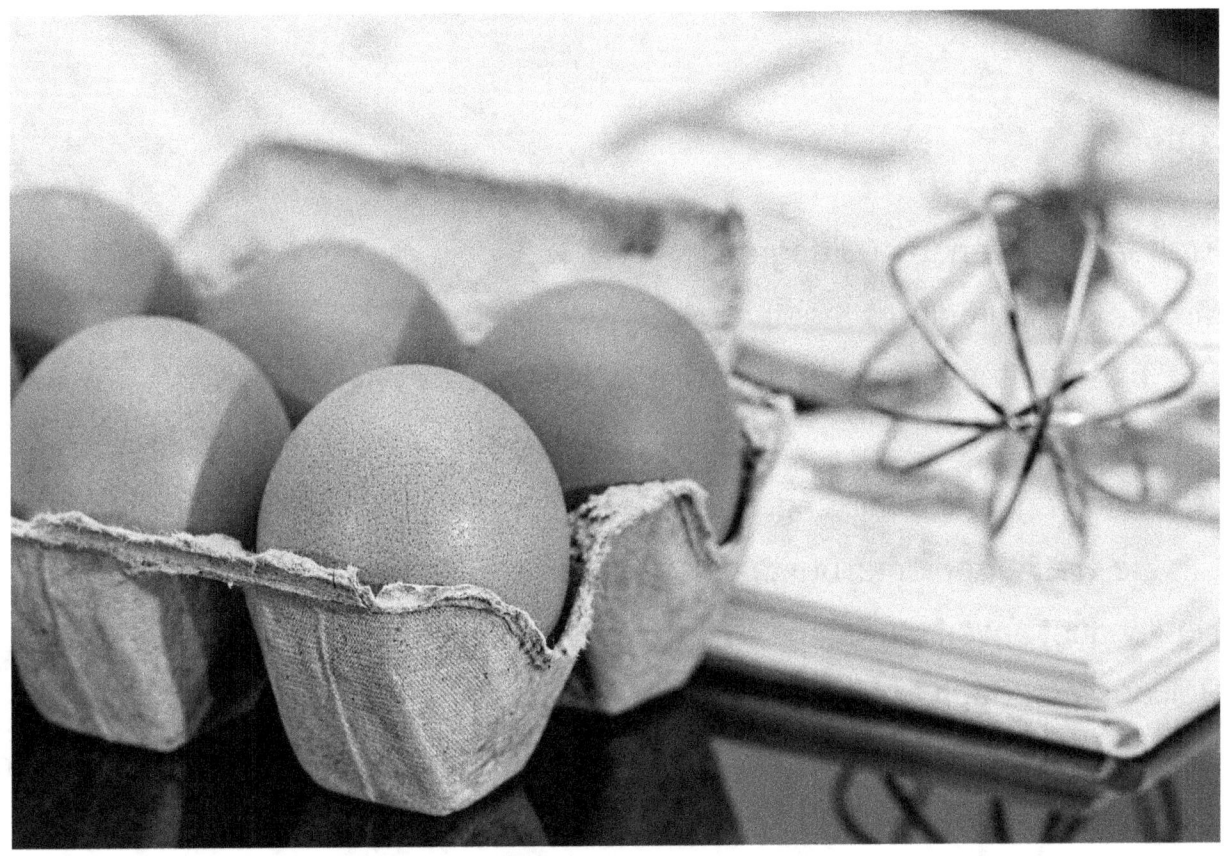

## Country Biscuits

Serves 8

Gluten free baking mixes have come so far in the last ten years. They are also now available in most grocery stores.

**Ingredients:**

3 ½ cups gluten free flour mix
¼ cup sugar
4 tsp. baking powder
1 tsp. salt
1 cup cold butter or buttery spread, cut up into small pieces

4 eggs
2/3 cup almond milk

**Directions:**

1. Preheat the oven to 400 degrees.
2. Mix the dry ingredients together.
3. Cut in the butter with a pastry cutter or dull knife, leaving some visible pieces of butter.
4. Whisk the eggs and milk together.
5. Stir the wet ingredients into the dry ingredients.
6. Lightly dust a work surface with flour or use parchment paper.
7. Roll out the dough to about ¾ inch thick.
8. Use a round cutter to make the biscuits, setting them about 2 inches apart on an ungreased cookie sheet.
9. Put the cookie sheet into the refrigerator for about 10 minutes to let the butter get cold again to help the biscuits to be flakey.
10. Bake the biscuits for about 15 minutes or until they are lightly brown.

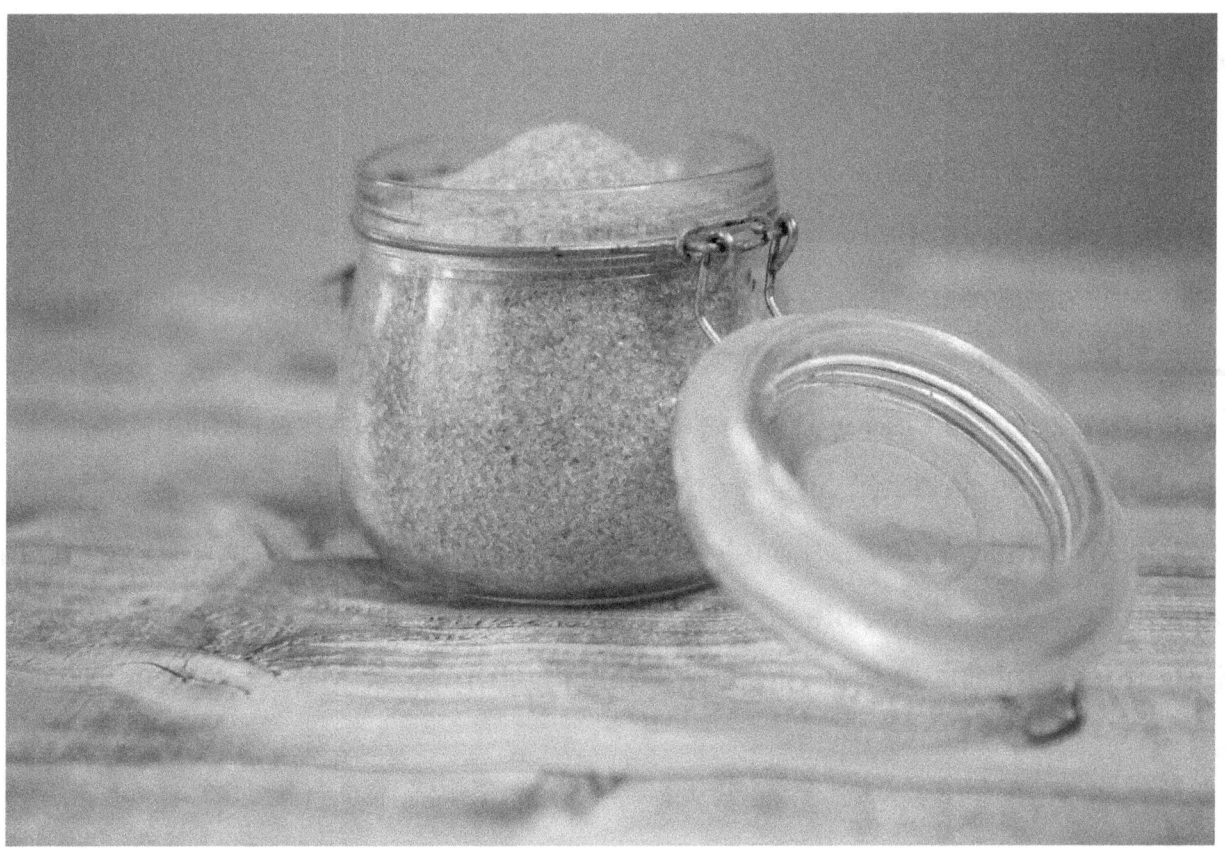

# Grilled Plantains with Brown Sugar Glaze

Serves 4

When my son's reflux was at its worst, plantains were one of the few foods he could tolerate. They have a relatively high pH and when cooked are easy to digest. Plantains are sweet and delicious and can be served as dessert or a side dish.

**Ingredients:**

3 Tbs. butter
¾ cup brown sugar
4 very ripe plantains (they will be almost black when ripe)

**Directions:**

1. Oil your grill or grill pan.
2. Preheat the grill too high.
3. In a small saucepan, mix the butter and sugar together. Heat the mixture on the stove top until the butter is melted. Remove from heat.
4. Slice the unpeeled plantains in half lengthwise and leave the peeling on.
5. Place them upside down on the grill (skin sides up).
6. Turn the plantains over and baste them with the butter and brown sugar mixture.
7. Cook for another 10 minutes. Brush with a bit more of the glaze.
8. Serve the plantains in their skins while still warm

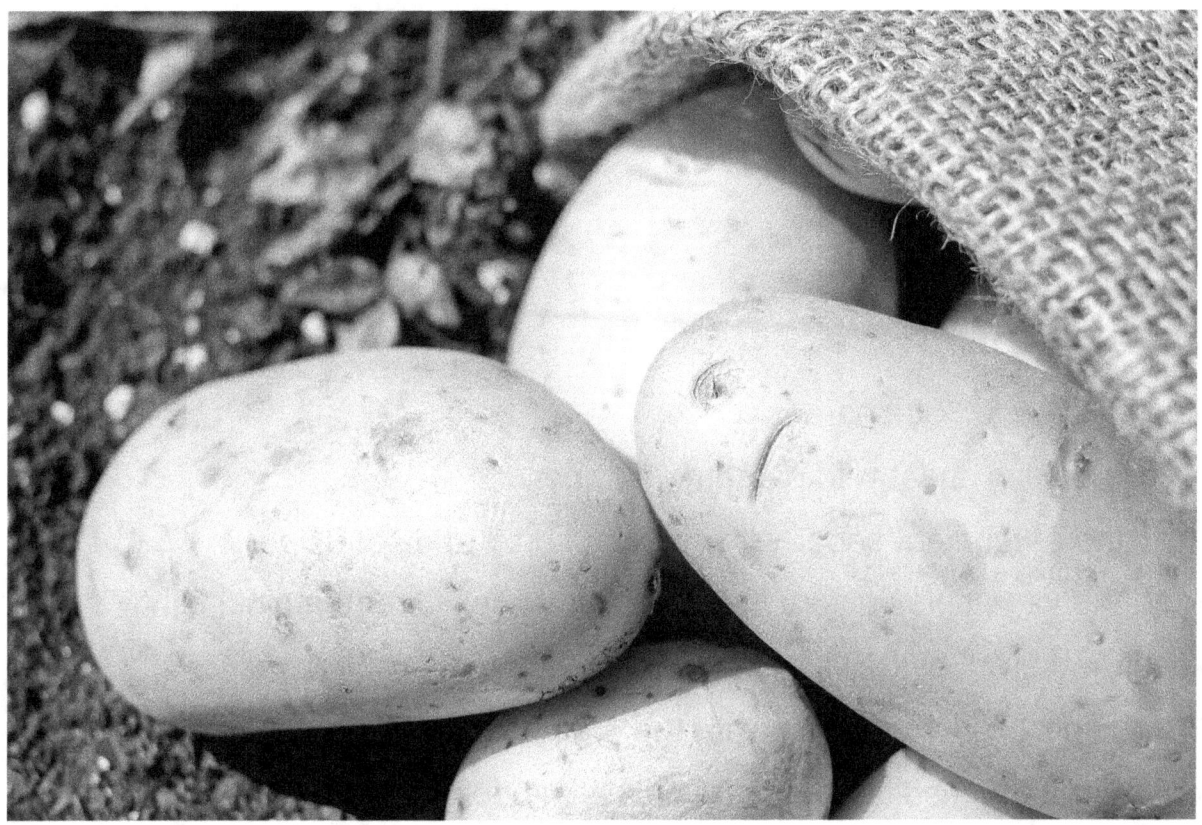

# Potato-Zucchini Latkes

Serves 4

White potatoes were one of the foods my son could tolerate so I was always searching for new ways to serve potatoes. The addition of the zucchini makes these extra moist and filled with vitamins and fiber. The applesauce topping makes them kid friendly.

**Ingredients:**

2 Yukon gold potatoes (shredded with a box grater)
1 medium zucchini (peeled and shredded)
1 onion (if tolerated) (chopped)

1 egg, lightly beaten
2 Tbs. flour (can substitute gluten free)
Salt and pepper to taste
Cooking spray
1 cup applesauce for serving

**Directions:**

1. Preheat oven to 350 degrees.
2. Cover a baking sheet with parchment paper.
3. Spray the parchment paper with cooking spray and set aside.
4. Shred the vegetables onto a clean kitchen towel. Over the sink, lightly squeeze the excess water out of the veggies.
5. Mix the shredded vegetables with the egg, flour, salt and pepper.
6. Heat a skillet to medium heat and coat with cooking spray.
7. Make the latkes into small patties and place in the skillet. Lightly brown each side just enough to keep their form.
8. Remove from the skillet and place on the baking sheet. Bake about 25 minutes – until the latkes are cooked through but not too dry). Serve warm with applesauce on top.

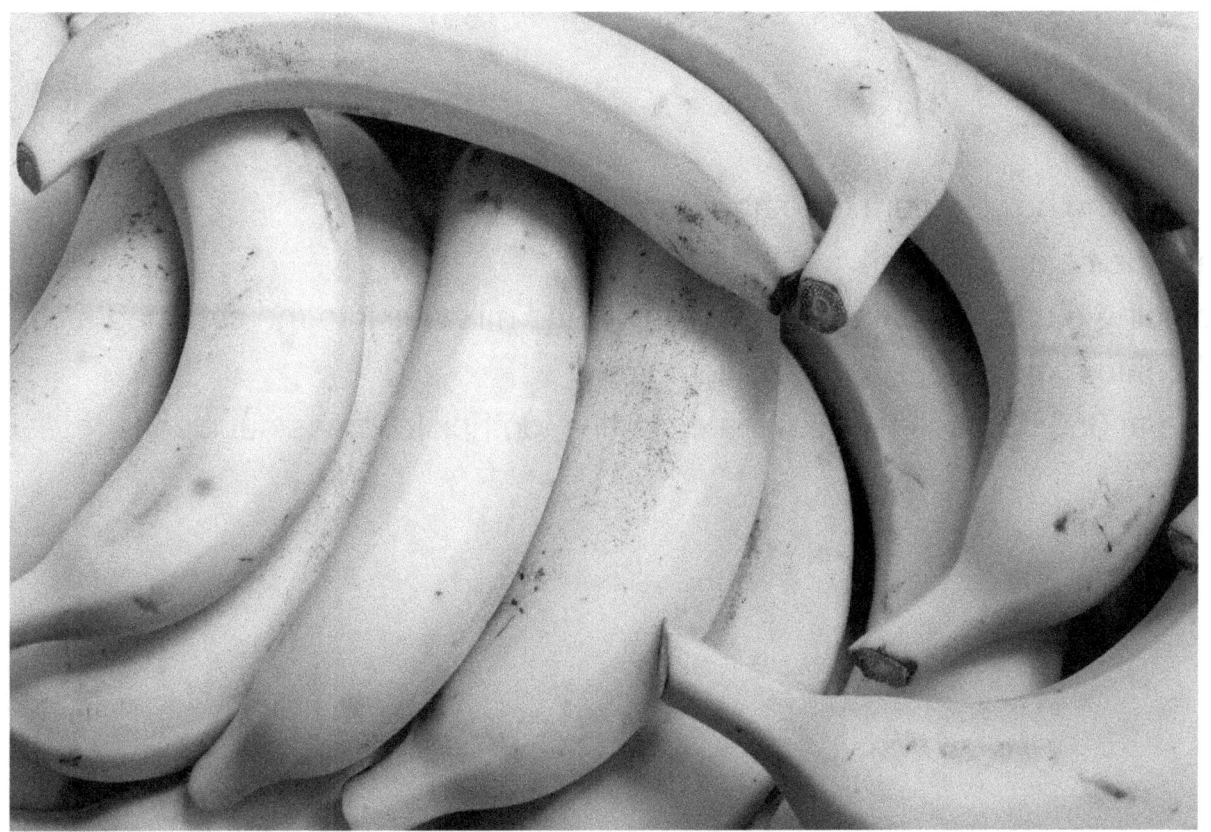

# Banana Bars

Serves 8

One of the things I learned early on with reflux friendly cooking is to keep the recipe as simple as possible. These bars are moist and delicious and will travel very well.

**Ingredients:**

½ cup butter
2 cups sugar
3 eggs
3 mashed ripe bananas
1 tsp. baking soda

½ tsp. salt

**Directions:**

1. In a mixing bowl, cream together the butter and sugar.
2. Beat the eggs, bananas and vanilla.
3. Combine the flour, baking soda, and salt and mix well into the creamed mixture.
4. Pour into a greased 9" x 13" baking pan.
5. Bake at 350 degrees for 25 minutes until a toothpick comes out clean.

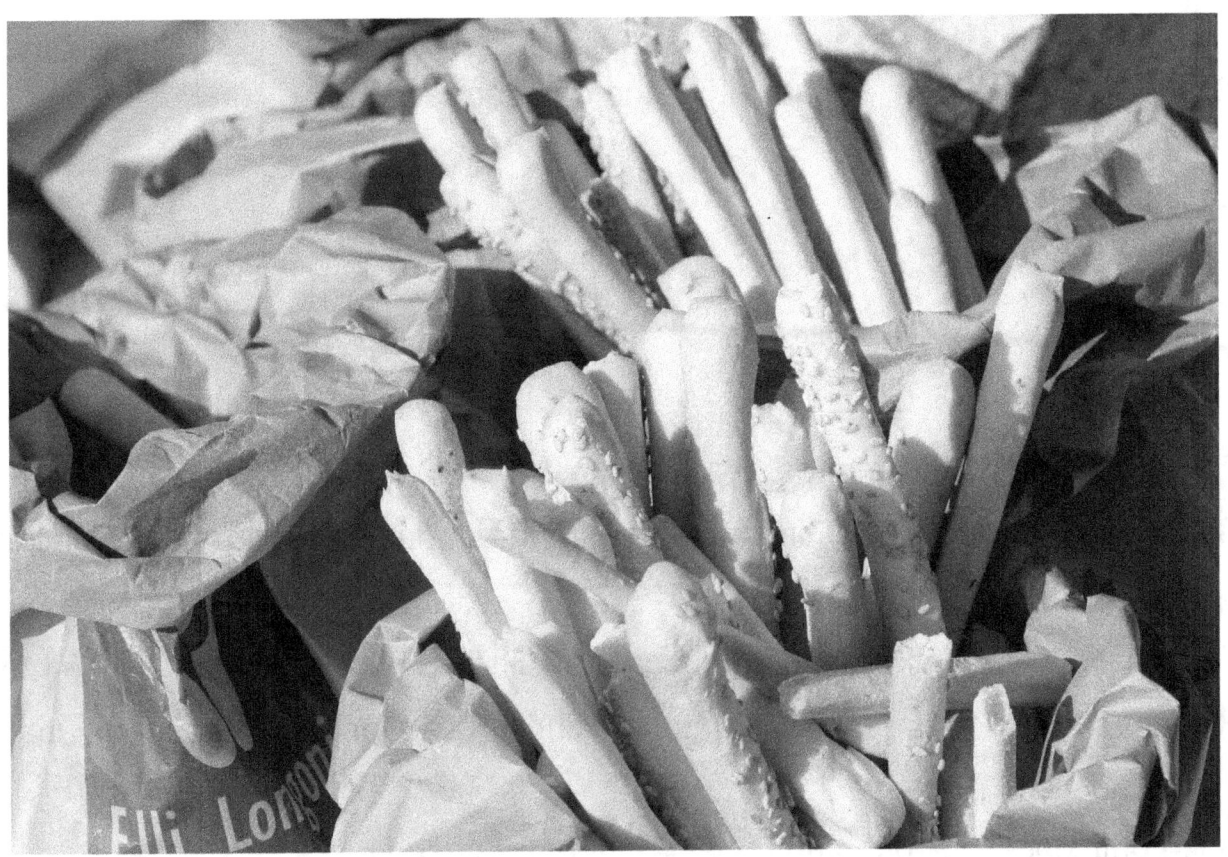

## Candied Bacon Sticks

Serves 8

One of my tricks when cooking reflux friendly food is to make it sound as fun and decadent as possible, while reducing as many triggers as possible. You will find when you are living a real life taking care of someone with reflux, you just cannot serve rice cakes 24/7. These breadsticks are beyond simple and make a wonderful appetizer for everyone.

**Ingredients:**

8 Italian breadsticks (they are usually in the cracker section)
Cooking spray
8 slices turkey bacon
1 cup brown sugar

**Directions:**

1. Preheat oven to 325 degrees.
2. Cover baking sheet in aluminum foil or parchment paper and spray with cooking spray.
3. Wrap each breadstick with turkey bacon, leaving an inch uncovered on both ends.
4. Place the wrapped breadsticks on the baking sheet. Sprinkle the brown sugar over the breadsticks.
5. Bake until bacon is crisp and browned, about 50 minutes.

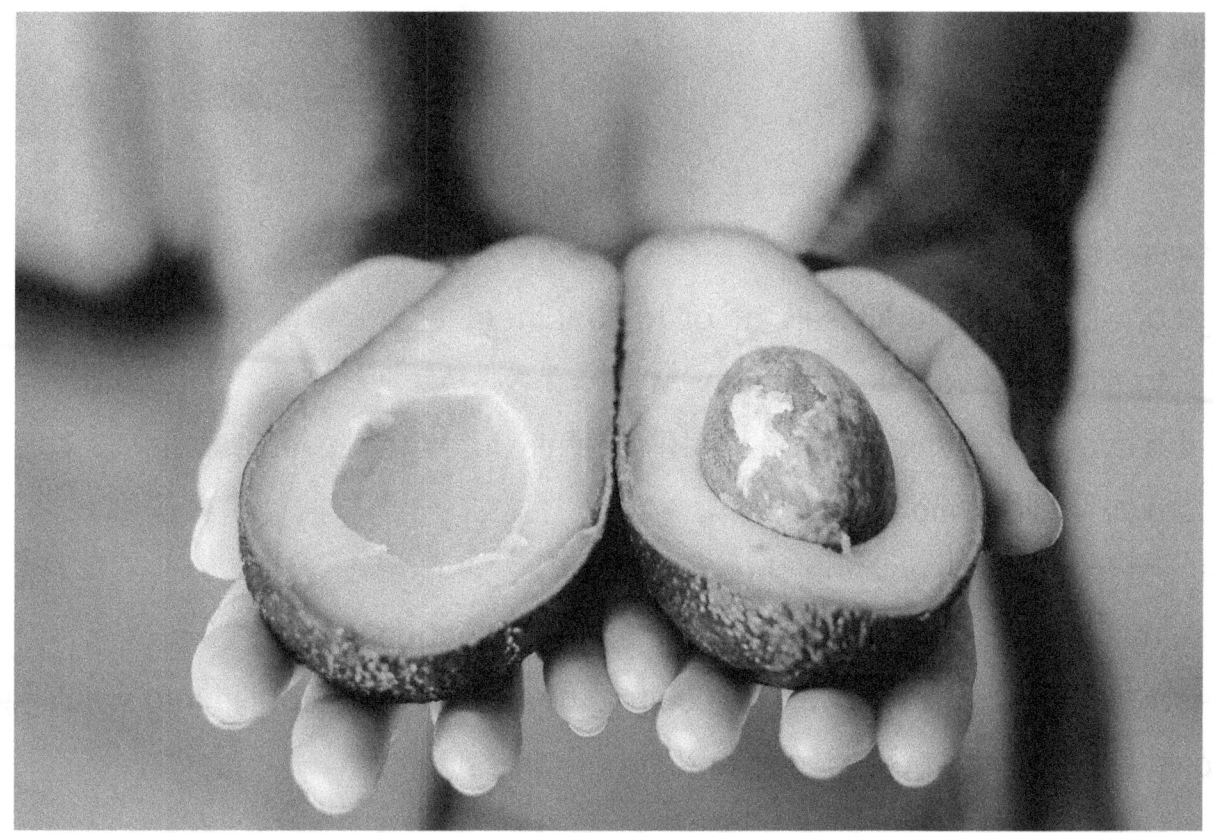

## Cheese Crispas with Avocado

Serves 4

Crispas were something they served at one of our favorite Mexican restaurants in Morgantown, West Virginia. However, since my son could not tolerate the spices and salsa in the real recipe, I recreated a reflux friendly version at home.

**Ingredients:**

4 medium or large tortillas (gluten free works fine)
½ cup olive oil
2 cups cheese (we used rice cheese)
2 ripe avocados, peeled and smashed
½ cup plain yogurt (dairy free works fine)

Salt and pepper to taste

**Directions:**

1. Preheat oven to 300 degrees.
2. In a large bowl, toss the tortillas in the oil to coat them.
3. Place the tortillas on two baking sheets.
4. Bake in the oven for 10 minutes, and then carefully turn them over.
5. Top the browned side with cheese.
6. Return them to the oven until the cheese is melted.
7. In a bowl, mix together the avocado, yogurt, salt and pepper.
8. Remove the tortillas from the oven to a cutting board. Cut each tortilla into small pie-like pieces. Drizzle with the avocado and yogurt dressing.

# Chapter Three: Sandwiches

One of the secrets to reflux friendly cooking is to take some of the traditional favorites and just make a few simple substitutions. When you cook this way, no one will feel deprived.

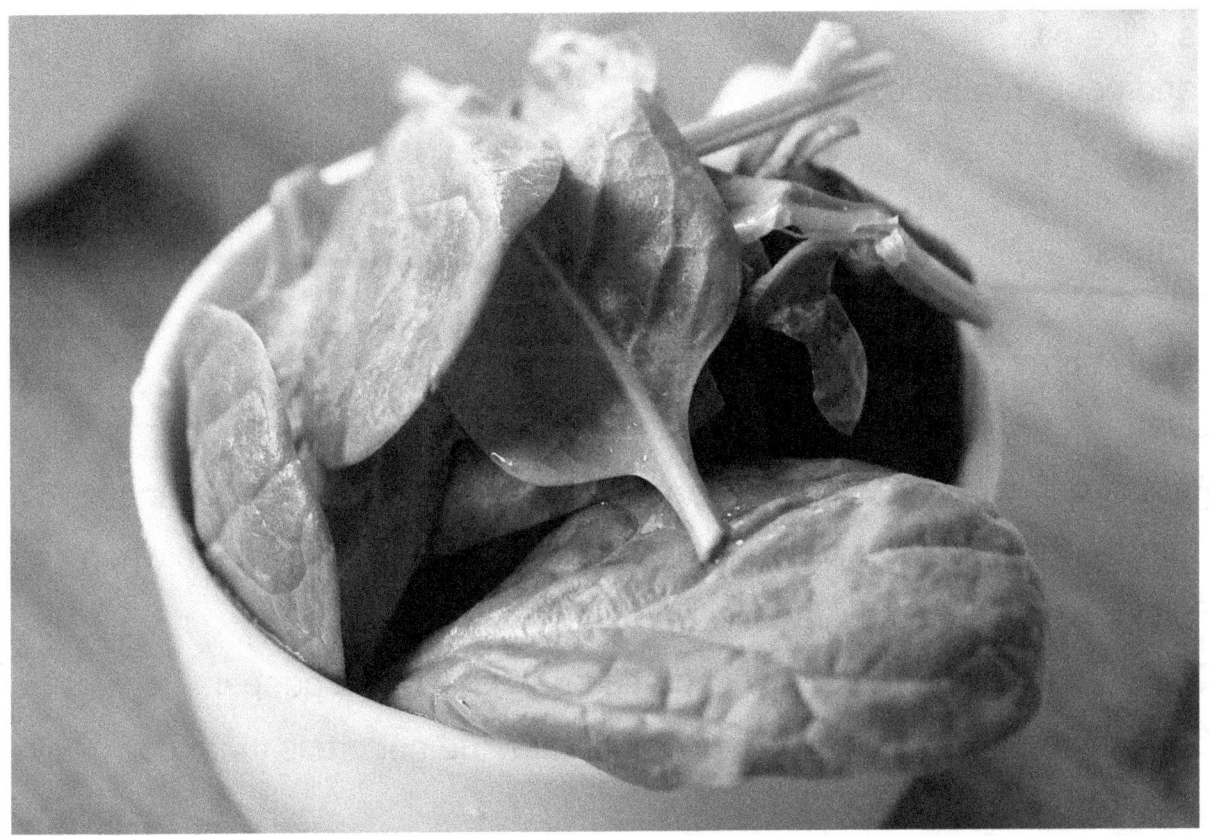

# California Burger

Serves 2

California cooking is all about fresh and colorful ingredients and this burger fits the bill.

**Ingredients:**

16 oz ground turkey
1 red pepper
1 avocado, sliced
1 cup baby spinach
1 Tbs. mayonnaise

2 hamburger buns (gluten free works fine)
2 slices cheese (non-dairy works fine)
1 Tbs. olive oil
Salt and pepper to taste
Cooking spray

**Directions:**

1. Lightly spray a cookie sheet with cooking spray.
2. Quarter a red pepper and remove the ribs and seeds.
3. Put the pepper on the cookie sheet and roast at 400 degrees for about 15 minutes
4. Remove the pepper from the oven and set aside. Slice into strips when cool.
5. Form the ground turkey into two patties.
6. Coat the burgers with olive oil and season with salt and pepper.
7. Cook the burgers in a skillet on medium heat (do not press them down with a spatula).
8. Turn once after about five minutes. Add the cheese just before they are done cooking.
9. Remove the patties and place on a paper towel to absorb any excess oil.
10. Place the burgers onto the buns coated with mayonnaise.
11. Top the burgers with avocado, spinach, and roasted red pepper.

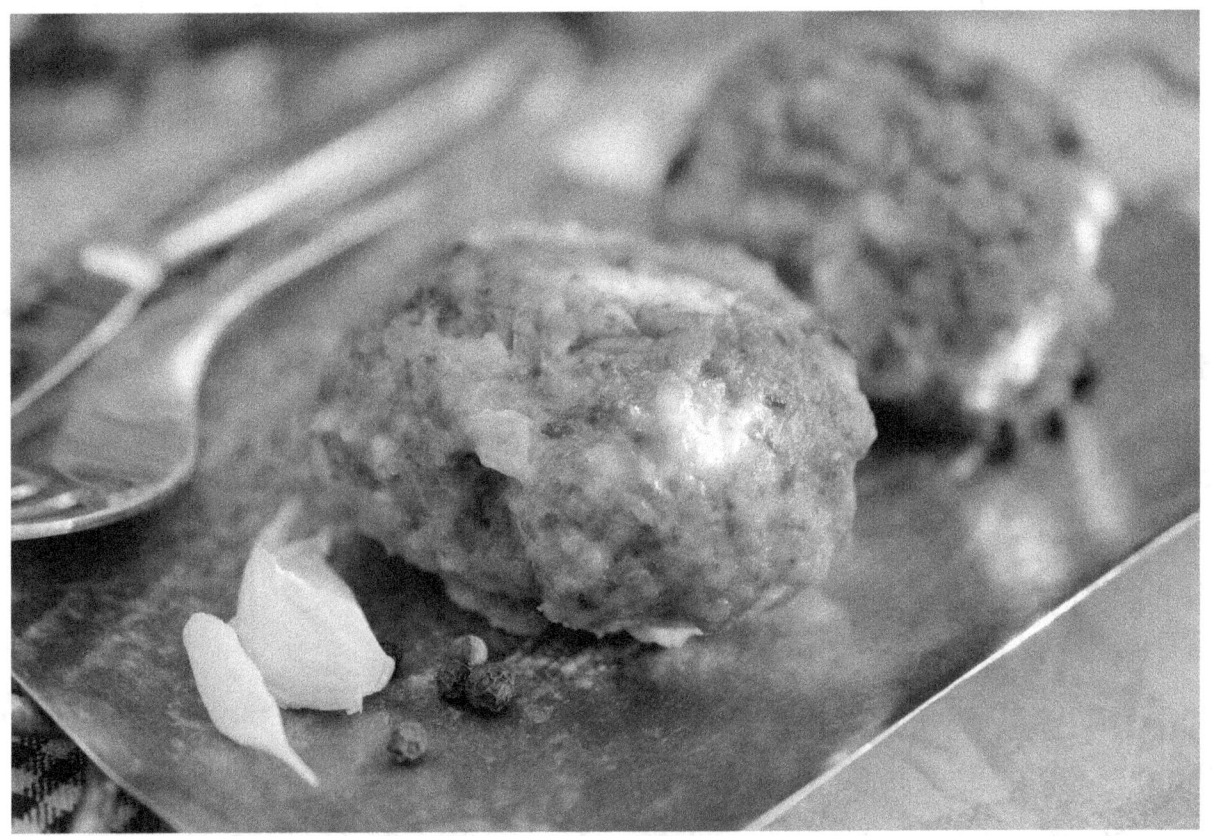

## Turkey Meatball Sub

Serves 2 or 3

Just because you have acid reflux, doesn't mean you don't crave big food. These meatball subs use a lower fat meatball and instead of an acidic barbecue sauce, they are topped with a less acidic roasted red pepper sauce.

**Ingredients:**

1 pound ground turkey
½ clove garlic (chopped fine)
½ cup bread crumbs (gluten free works fine)

¼ cup fresh parsley (minced)
1 large egg
2 tsp. Worcestershire sauce
Salt and pepper to taste
¼ cup olive oil
1 red pepper
1 cup mayonnaise
2 sub rolls (gluten free works fine)

**Directions:**

1. Lightly spray a cookie sheet with cooking spray.
2. Quarter a red pepper and remove the ribs and seeds.
3. Put the pepper on the cookie sheet and roast at 400 degrees for about 15 minutes.
4. Remove the pepper from the oven and let cool.
5. In a food processor or blender, mix the mayonnaise and red pepper. Set aside.
6. Combine the ground turkey, garlic, bread crumbs, parsley, egg, Worcestershire sauce, salt and pepper.
7. Roll into medium sized meatballs.
8. Add olive oil to skillet and heat to medium.
9. Cook meatballs, gently turning over as the brown. Cook approximately 10 minutes, until meatballs are cooked through but not dry.
10. Place meatballs on sub rolls and top with roasted red pepper sauce.

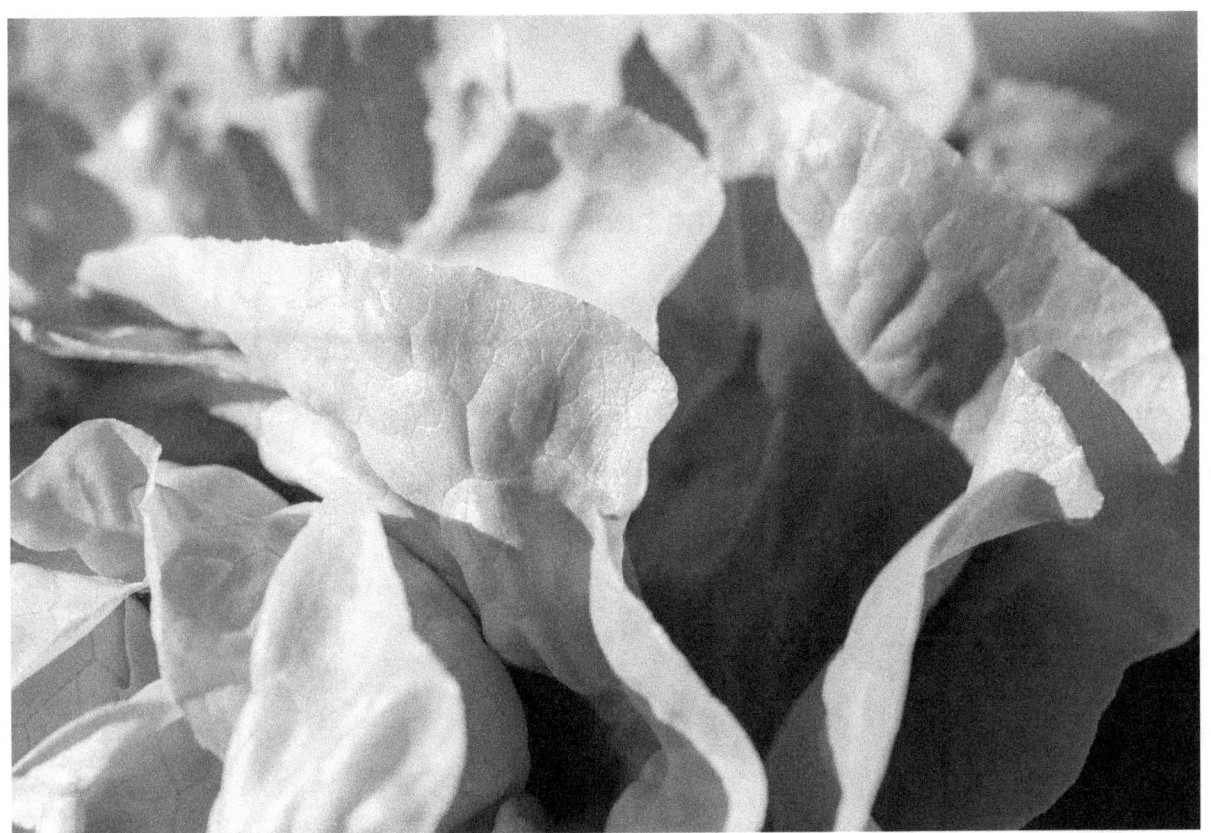

## Tuna Salad Lettuce Wrap

Serves 2

Tuna is extremely low fat and bib lettuce is a great way to ditch the bread if you are gluten free.

**Ingredients:**

4 pieces of bib lettuce
1 can of tuna (5 oz)
½ cup of mayonnaise
2 sticks celery (chopped)
Pinch of salt and pepper to taste

**Directions:**

1. Rinse the lettuce with cool water and let dry.
2. Remove the lettuce leaves from the bunch so they each stay intact.
3. Drain the tuna.
4. In a bowl, mix together the tuna, mayonnaise, celery, salt and pepper.
5. Lay each lettuce leaf in your hand and fill the middle with ¼ of the tuna salad.
6. Fold the lettuce over gently and keep refrigerated before serving.

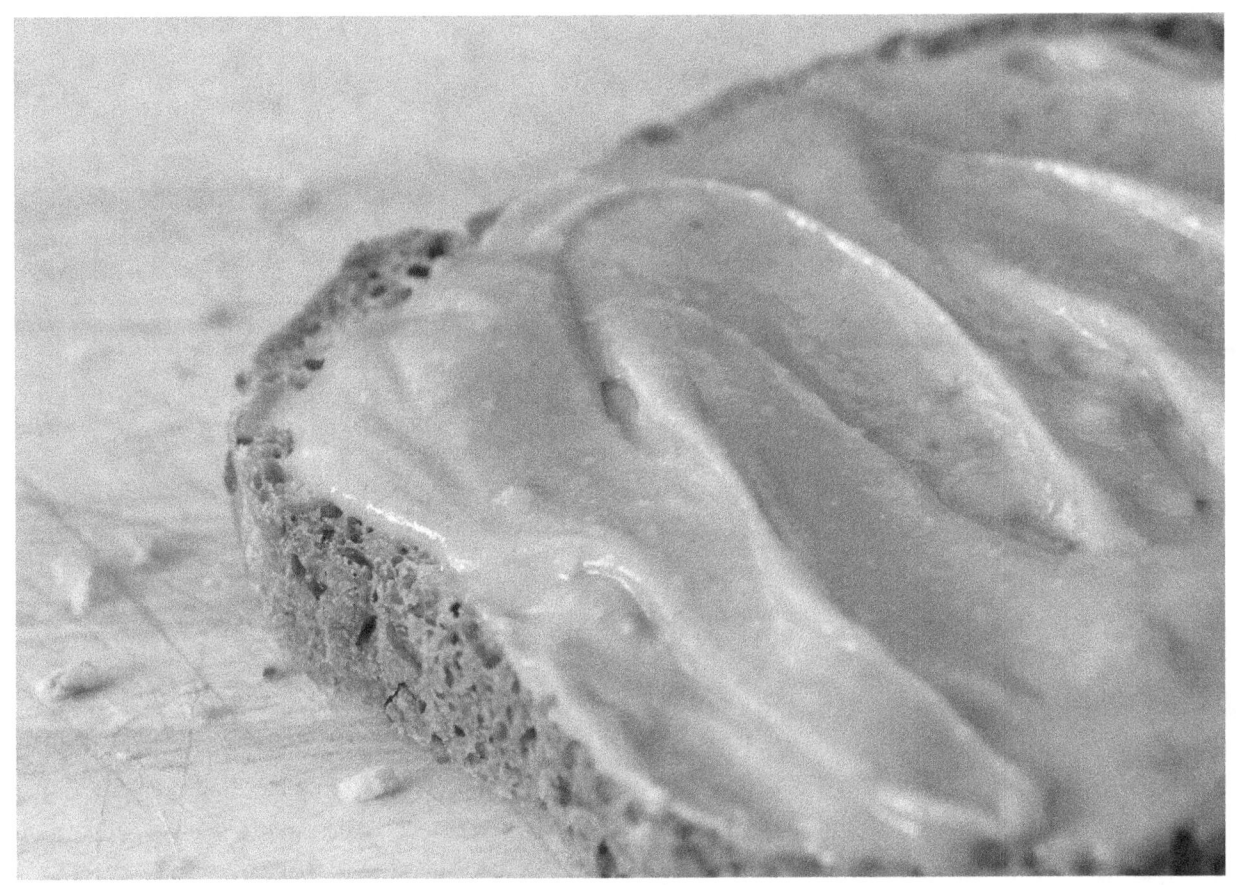

# Almond Butter, Banana and Honey Sandwich

Serves 1

Almond butter is made from grinding almonds into nut butter. Almond butter is a nice alternative to peanut butter and is full of vitamins and minerals. Bananas are low acidic and the combination can be gentle on the stomach.

Ingredients:
2 slices bread
2 Tbs. almond butter
½ banana, sliced

1 Tbs. honey

Directions:
Top the bread with almond butter, bananas, and honey.

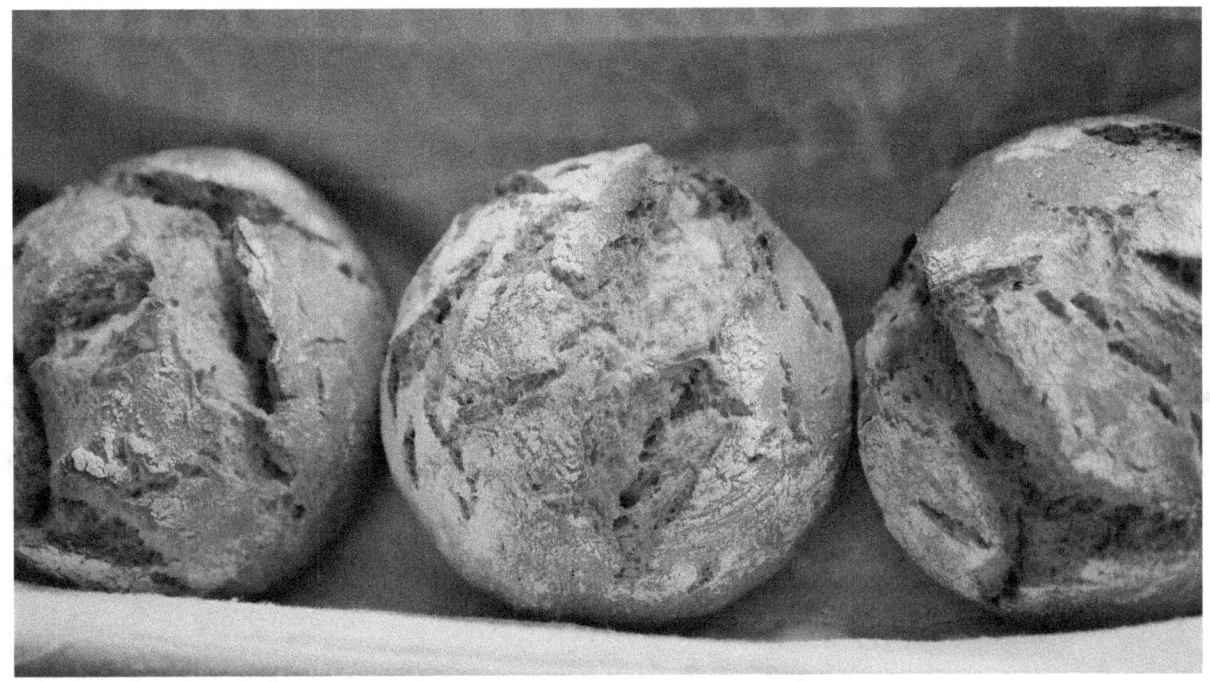

# Grilled Turkey Reuben

Serves 1

This sandwich is a riff on a standard Reuben sandwich. Substituting turkey for the corned beef can reduce the fat content and using coleslaw instead of sauerkraut can make it less acidic.

**Ingredients:**

½ cup coleslaw
5 ounces of sliced turkey
1 Tbs. butter
2 slices rye bread
2 slices Swiss cheese
2 Tbs. thousand island salad dressing

**Directions:**

1. Spread butter generously on one side of each slice of rye bread, then spread the thousand island dressing on the other side.
2. Top the thousand island side with coleslaw, turkey, and Swiss cheese. Top with the other slice of bread, butter-side up.
3. Heat a large skillet over medium-low heat. Arrange the sandwich on the skillet and grill until lightly browned and the cheese is melted, about 3 minutes on each side.

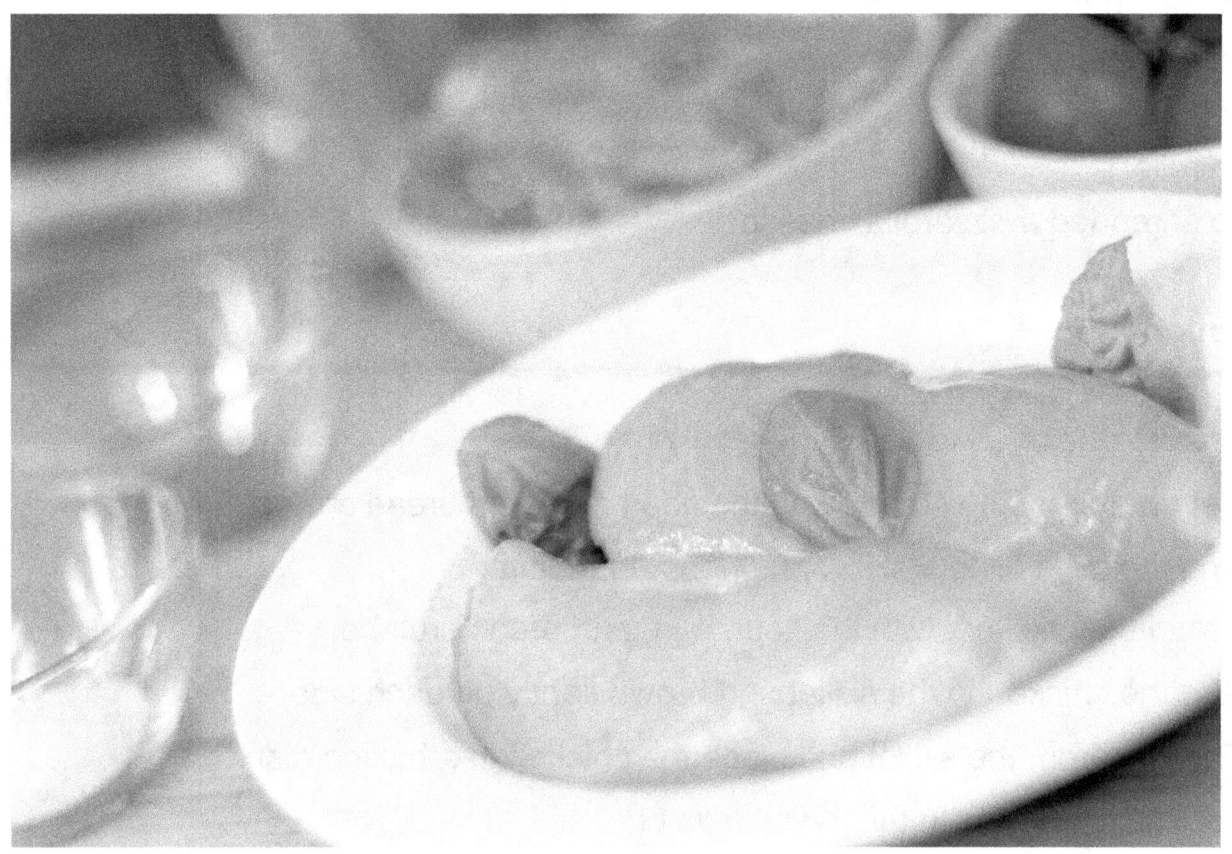

# Chicken Parmesan Sub

Serves 2

I still make chicken parmesan for my son almost every week. One of the great things about this recipe is that you can customize each sub to match your needs.

**Ingredients**:

2 chicken breasts, butterflied open with a sharp knife
1 cup flour
1 egg, beaten slightly

1 cup panko bread crumbs
2 Tbs. olive oil
½ cup mayonnaise
2 sub rolls
1 cup shredded mozzarella cheese

**Directions:**

1. Preheat the oven to 350 degrees.
2. Set up a breading station with the flour, egg, and bread crumbs.
3. Add the olive oil to a skillet and heat to medium.
4. Bread the chicken, with the flour, egg, and bread crumbs.
5. Add the chicken to the skillet and brown lightly on each side.
6. Remove from the skillet and place the chicken in a baking dish.
7. Top the chicken with the mozzarella cheese.
8. Finish baking the chicken in oven, depending on the thickness, for about 15 minutes.
9. Spread the sub rolls with mayonnaise and top with the chicken breasts. Serve warm.

# Chapter Four: Entrees

Managing reflux involves eating smaller, more frequent meals. However, if you are cooking for a family, you still need to make dinners that sound heavy but are light and easily digestible. The recipes below are just right.

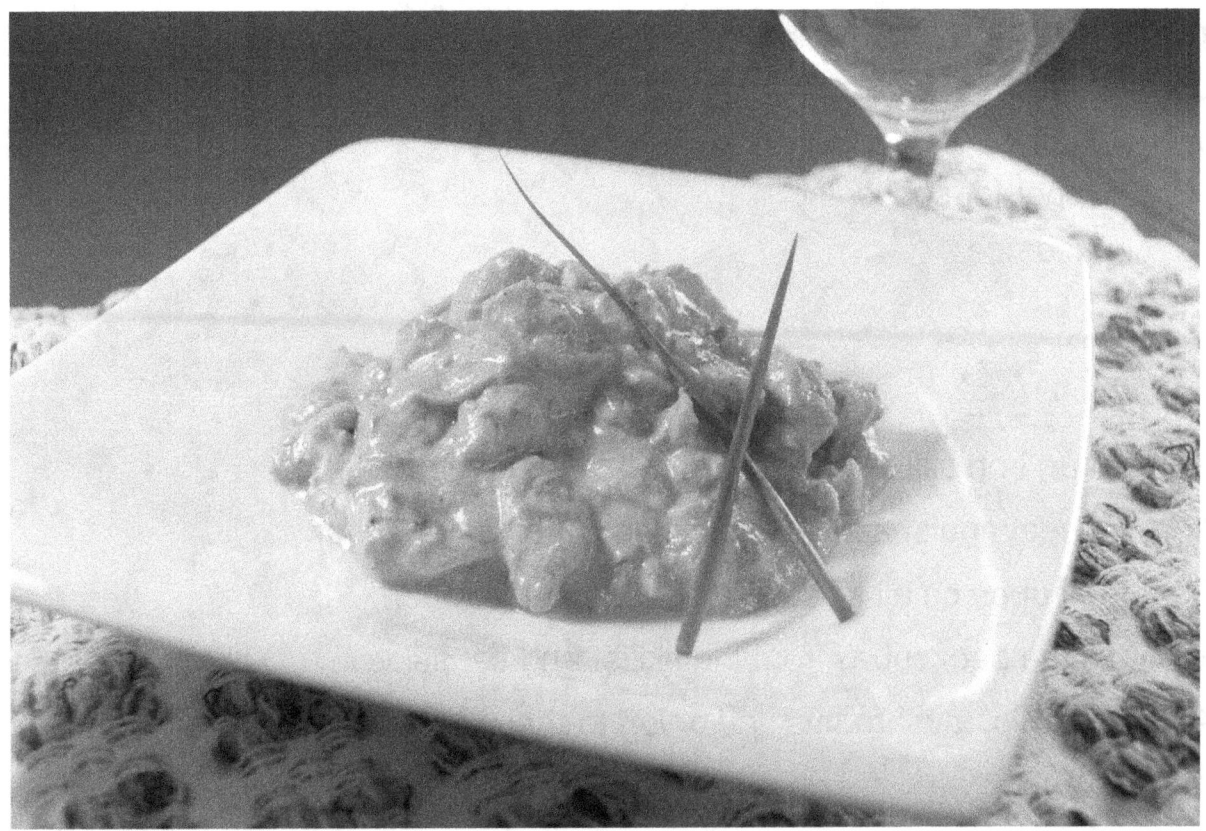

# Beef Stroganoff

Serves 2

This dish can be extremely comforting, but the traditional recipe can be too heavy for someone with acid reflux disease. However, with a few modifications, you can turn this classic into a gluten free, dairy free, and reflux friendly meal that everyone can enjoy.

**Ingredients**:

1 Tbs. olive oil
1 lb. sirloin steak, cut into cubes
1 clove garlic, minced

1 package button mushrooms, cut in half
½ onion, diced
¾ cup beef broth
2 Tbs. oat flour
Salt and pepper for seasoning
2 cups cooked rice

**Directions**:

1. Preheat an iron skillet to medium and add the oil.
2. Add the beef and season with a pinch of salt and pepper.
3. Sear the cubes on all sides, but do not cook through.
4. Remove the beef cubes from the skillet and set aside.
5. Add the garlic, mushrooms and onion to the skillet and sauté until the onion is transparent.
6. Return the beef to the skillet and sprinkle in the oat flour.
7. Add the beef broth, stir to combine and simmer until the beef is cooked through, but not over cooked.

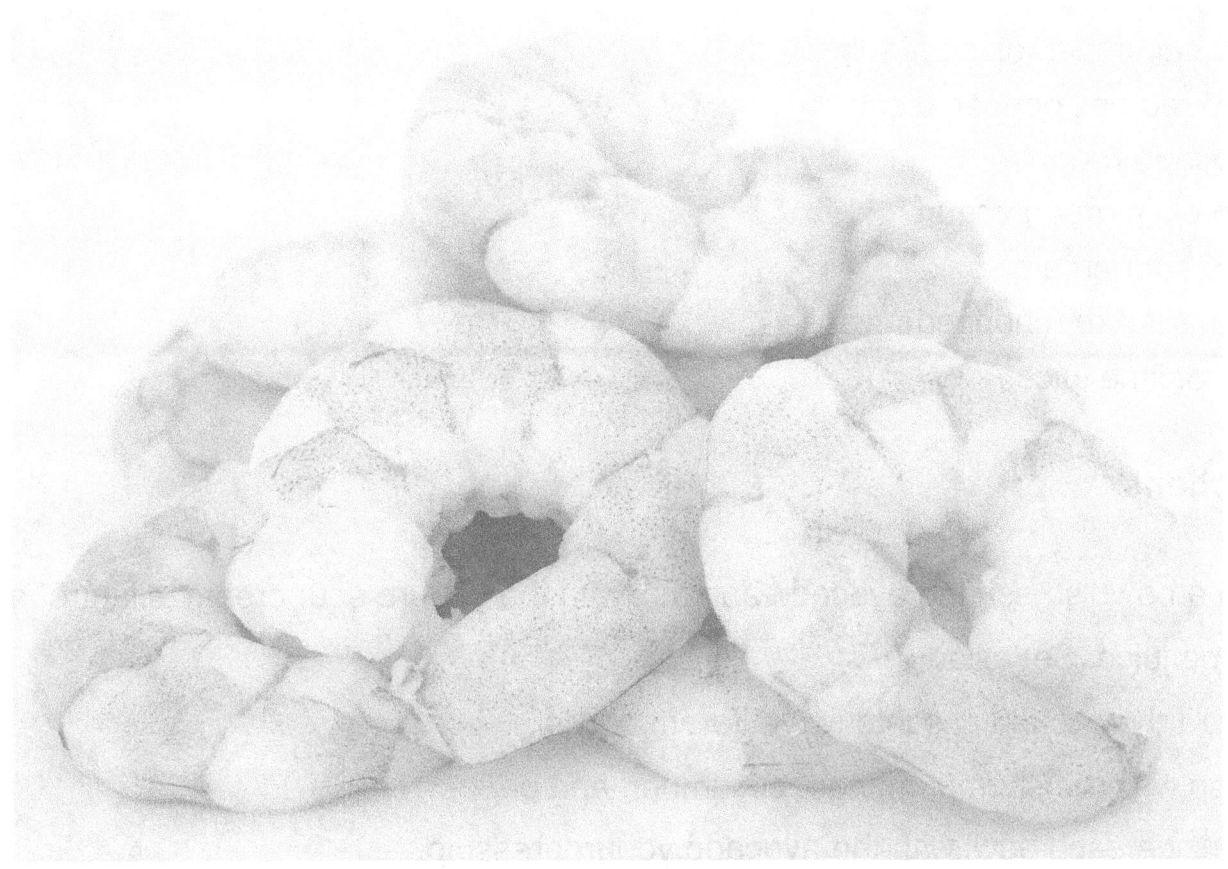

# Shrimp Poke Bowls

Serves 2

Poke bowls are a Hawaiian dish and every time I make them I am transported to the tropics. One of the great things about these bowls is you can make easy substitutions based on what you tolerate the best.

**Ingredients**:

1 bag instant rice, cooked and chilled
1 dozen shrimp, peeled, cooked, and chilled

1 cup fresh mango, diced
1 cup cucumber, diced (if tolerated)
½ cup red bell pepper, diced
1 avocado (ripe)
1 cup plain green yogurt
½ cup sour cream
1 Tbs. cilantro (chopped)
Dash of lime juice

**Directions**:

1. In a bowl, smash the avocado and mix with the yogurt, sour cream, cilantro, and lime juice. Set aside.
2. Split the cooked rice into two different bowls.
3. Top with the shrimp, mango, cucumber, and pepper.
4. Drizzle each bowl with the avocado yogurt dressing.
5. Serve cold.

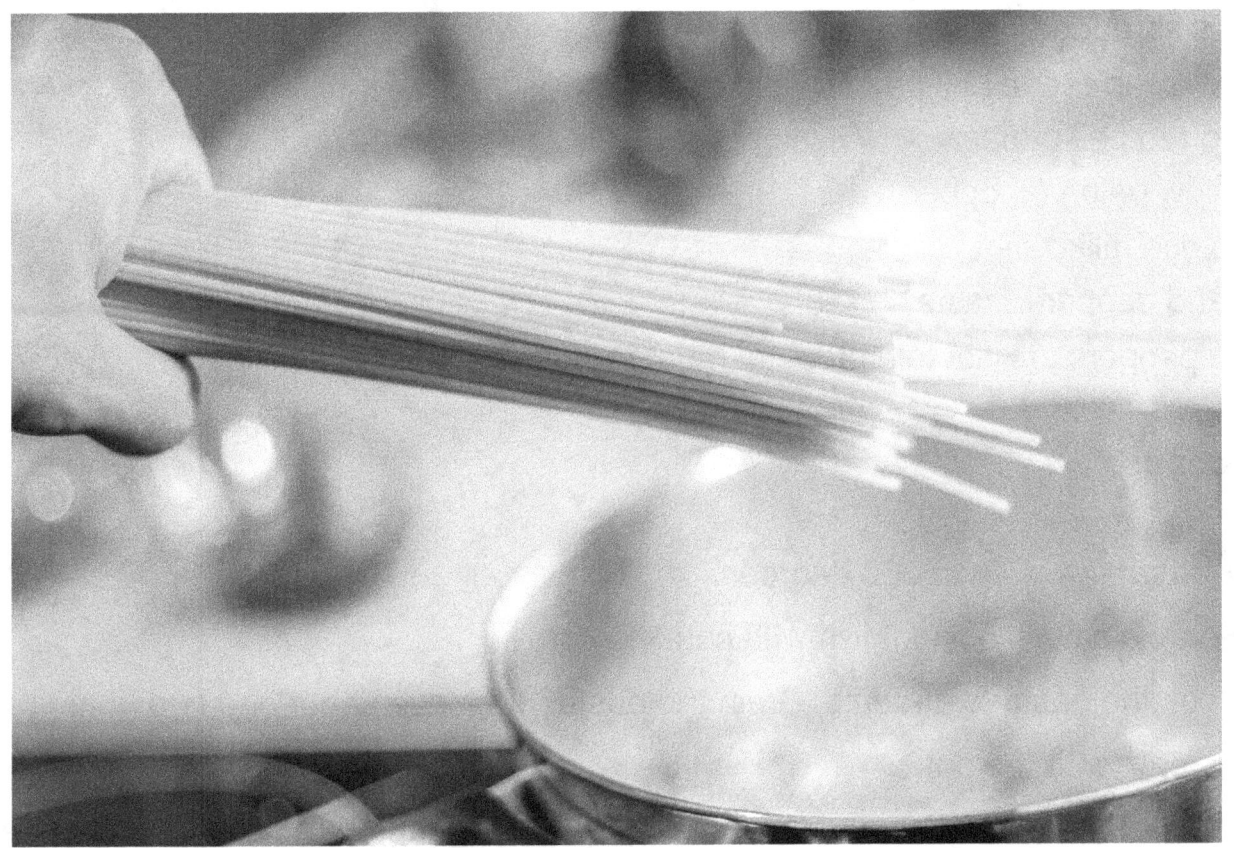

## Chicken Spaghetti

Serves 3 to 4

As you have probably figured out, acid reflux comes in waves. When acid reflux is at its worst, you have to really try as hard as you can to just get yourself or your child back on track. This recipe is gluten free and dairy free, but can still feel like you are enjoying a meal.

**Ingredients:**

Cooking spray
2 cups cooked chicken (diced)

½ package rice spaghetti (the pieces broken in half)
2 cups shredded rice cheese
¼ cup diced green bell pepper (if tolerated)
¼ cup red bell pepper
¼ yellow onion (chopped)
1 cup rice milk
Salt and pepper to taste
(if the peppers are not tolerated, try mushrooms and celery)

**Directions:**

1. Preheat the oven to 350 degrees.
2. Spray a small cooking dish with cooking spray.
3. Cook the pasta to al-dente. Drain the pasta, but leave about one cup of hot pasta water in with the pot.
4. Add the chicken, peppers, onion, salt, pepper, milk and one cup of the cheese to the pot. Gently mix together. Pour the pasta mixture into the baking dish.
5. Top the pasta with the other cup of cheese.
6. Cover with foil and bake for 30 minutes.
7. Serve warm.

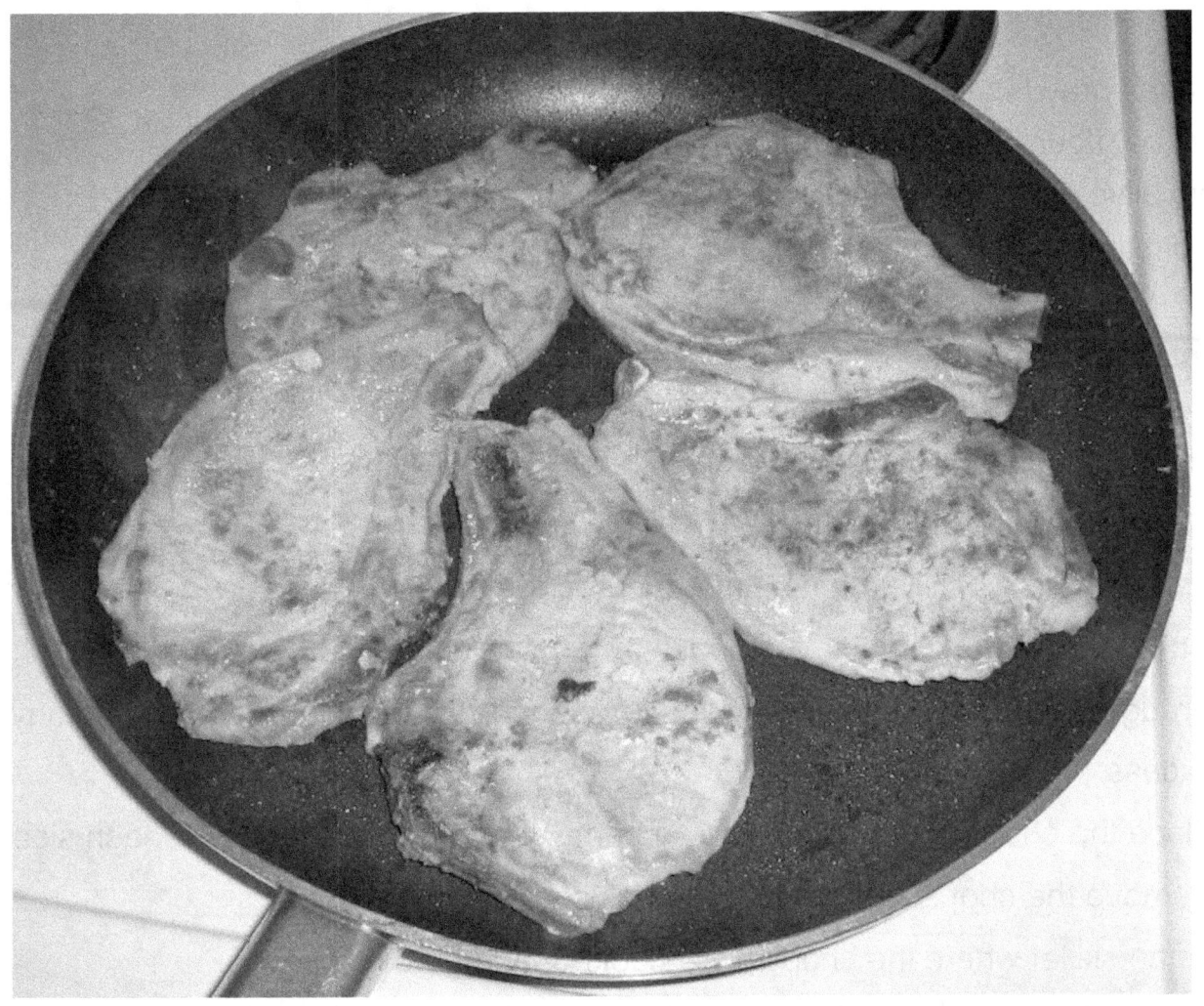

# Pork Chops with Gravy

Serves 4

One way to curb the cravings of heavier food is to meet the cravings half way by making a recipe that sounds heavy but is really reflux friendly. Pork chops are known as the "other white meat" and can be a lower fat alternative to red meat.

**Ingredients**:

Cooking spray, 4 thinly cut pork chops (with or without bone in)
¾ cup oat flour, Salt and pepper to taste
2 Tbs. olive oil, 2 Tbs. oat flour
¼ cup milk (non-dairy milk works fine)

**Directions**:

1. Lightly coat a shallow baking dish with cooking spray.
2. Preheat oven to 300 degrees.
3. Preheat a large skillet on medium and add the olive oil.
4. On a large plate, combine the flour, salt and pepper.
5. Dredge each side of the pork chops through the flour mixture, shaking off any excess.
6. Place the chops in the skillet. Brown briefly – about two minutes on each side.
7. Remove the chops and place in the baking pan.
8. In the skillet where the chops were cooked, add 2 Tbs. flour.
9. Stir the flour constantly for about 30 seconds.
10. Add the milk (starting with 1/8 cup) and continue stirring on medium low heat until gravy thickens (if the gravy is too thick, you can add more milk slowly).
11. Add a pinch of salt and pepper for flavor.
12. Remove the gravy from the heat and spoon on top of the pork chops. Cover the pork chops in foil and bake for 15 minutes.
13. Uncover and bake for another 15 minutes (or until fork tender, but do not overcook).
14. Serve warm with rice or potatoes.

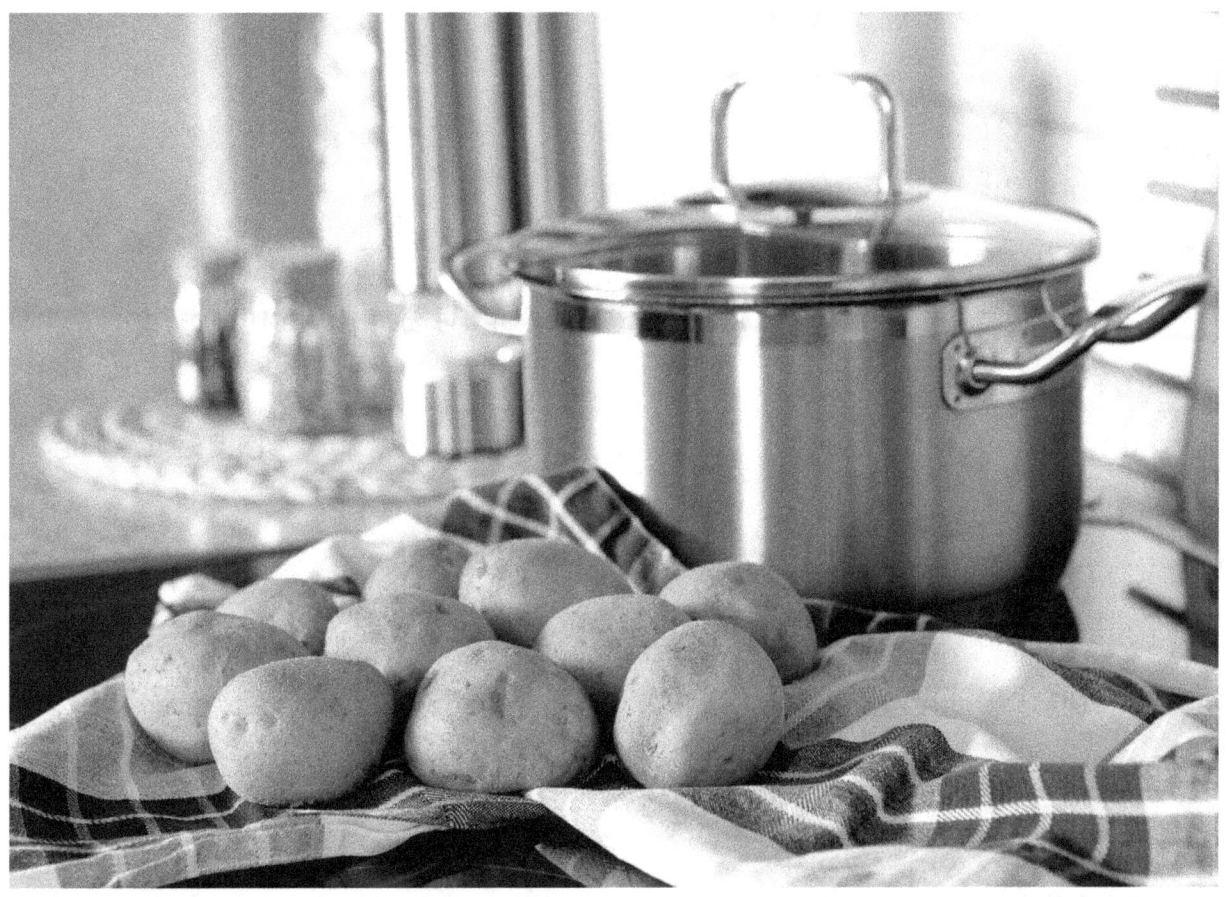

# Creamy Potato Soup

Serves 2

It can be hard to find a soup that is not tomato-based or loaded with fat. This soup is comforting, low fat, and easy to digest.

**Ingredients**:

Two medium white potatoes
2 cups rice milk
1 cup rice cheese

Salt and pepper to taste

**Directions**:

1. Peel and boil the potatoes until fork tender.
2. Remove from heat and cut into chunks.
3. In a blender, add the rice milk. Then add half of the potato chunks, half of the cheese, salt, and pepper.
4. Blend until smooth (be careful to allow steam to escape your blender while blending).
5. Pour the blended soup into a bowl.
6. Add the other half of the potato chunks.
7. Top with the remaining cheese.
8. Serve warm.

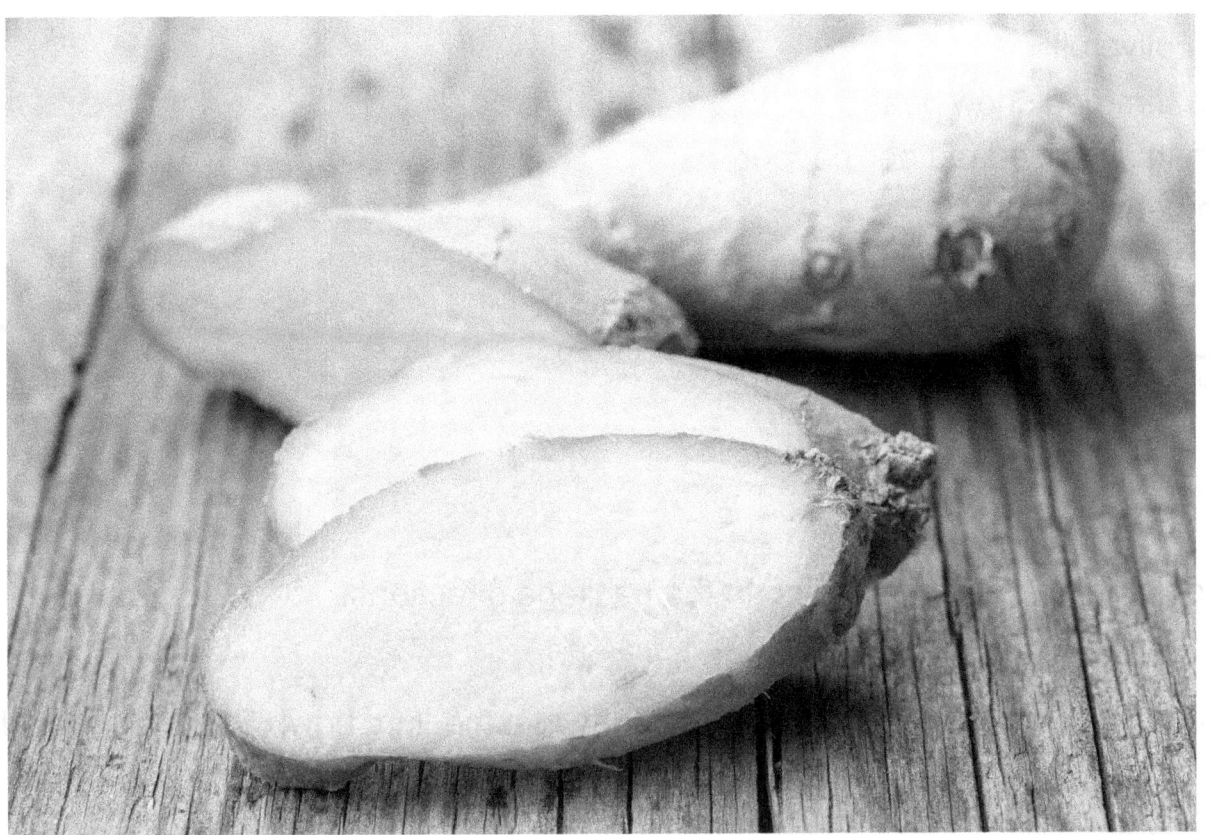

# Shrimp Lo Mein

Serves 2 or 3

Chinese take-out often contains more fat and spice than most with reflux can tolerate. Instead of ordering out for the new year, try making this Asian-inspired dish at home.

**Ingredients**:

16 large peeled shrimp
8 oz spaghetti (gluten free works fine)
¼ cup chicken or vegetable stock
2 Tbs. soy sauce

1 Tbs. honey
2 Tbs. olive oil
½ cup trimmed snow peas
½ cup thinly sliced red bell pepper
1 cup bean sprouts
1 clove garlic, minced (if tolerated)
1 Tbs. minced fresh ginger
2 Tbs. sesame seeds

**Directions**:

1. Cook the spaghetti according to the package directions.
2. Drain and rinse under cold water, set aside.
3. Combine the broth, soy sauce and honey in a medium bowl. Stir and set aside.
4. Heat olive oil in a large skillet over medium heat.
5. Add the snow peas, bell pepper, bean sprouts, garlic, ginger and shrimp.
6. Sauté for 2 minutes or until the shrimp are pink, but not overcooked.
7. Add the broth mixture to the skillet and simmer the ingredients about 3 minutes or until heated through. Add the pasta and toss to combine.
8. Transfer to a serving bowl and sprinkle with the sesame seeds.

# Chapter Five: Desserts

When acid reflux disease first entered my world, I struggled with making desserts. I was unsure how to make a dessert that tasted good without high amounts of fat and chocolate. But with some work, I figured it out. Here are some of my favorites.

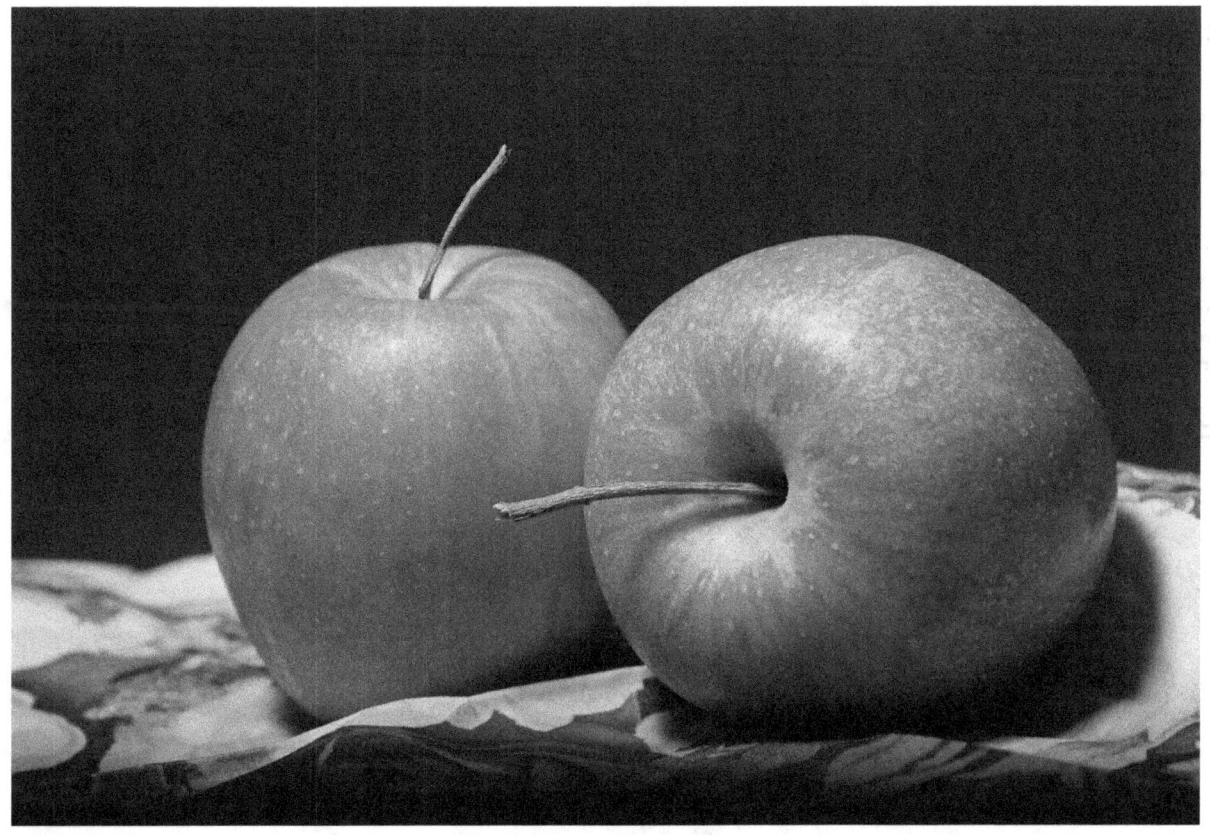

# Autumn's Apple Cake

Makes 2 loaf pans

**Ingredients**:

3 cups all-purpose flour (gluten free will work fine)
2 cups sugar
1 tsp. ground ginger
1 tsp. baking powder
1 ¼ cups canola oil
1 tsp. vanilla
2 eggs
3 medium apples (peeled, cored, and diced)

1 cup chopped pecans
1 cup raisins

**Directions**:

1. Preheat oven to 350 degrees.
2. Mix the dry ingredients together.
3. Then mix the eggs, oil, and vanilla and add to the dry ingredients.
4. Fold in the apples, raisins, and pecans.
5. Split the mix between two greased loaf pans.
6. Bake for one hour or until a toothpick comes out clean.
7. Let cool before cutting.

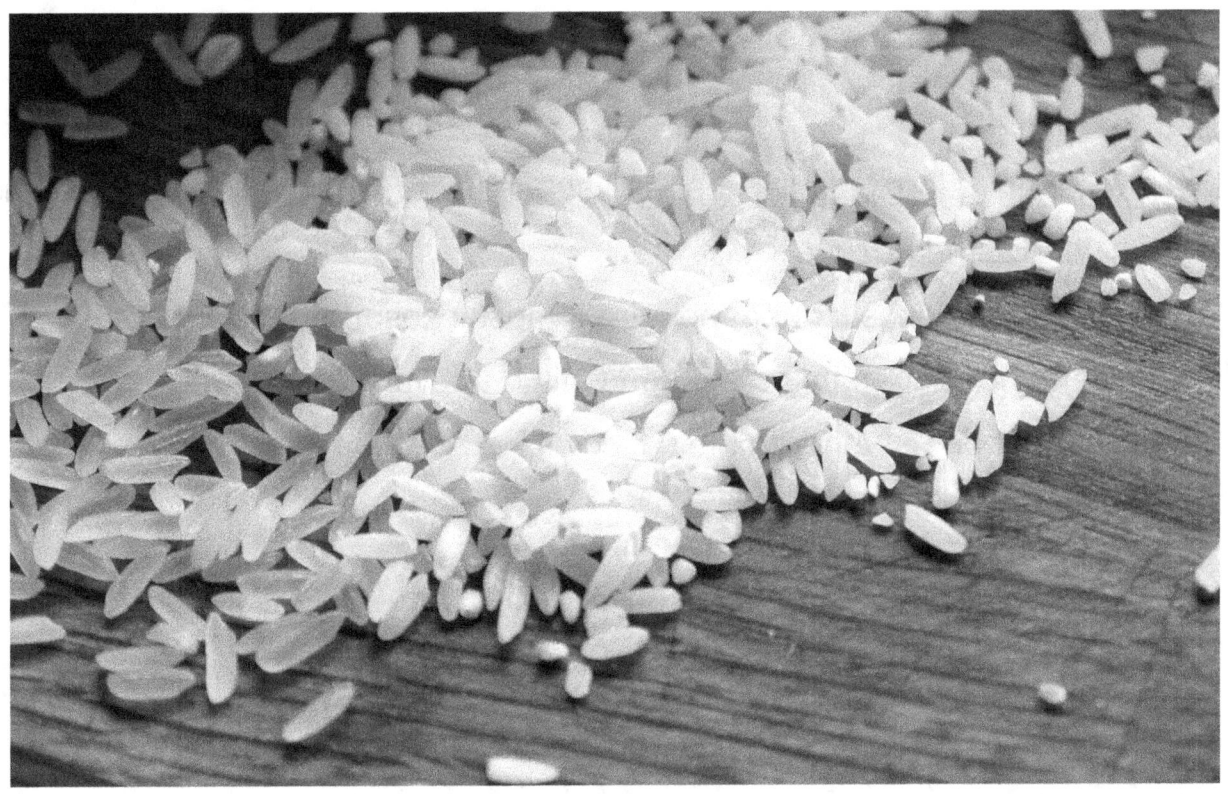

## Cool Rice Pudding

Serves 4

Rice pudding has always been a soothing treat for my son with acid reflux disease. The coconut milk in this recipe provides a healthy fat and the cashews add protein.

**Ingredients**:

4 cups coconut milk
½ cup basmati rice
3 Tbs. granulated sugar
1 tsp. pure vanilla extract
¼ tsp. salt

½ cup cashews

**Directions**:

1. In a saucepan, bring the milk, rice, and sugar just to a boil, immediately reducing the heat and stirring frequently.
2. Simmer until the rice is tender and milk is mostly absorbed (about 20-25 minutes).
3. Remove the pudding from the heat and stir in the vanilla and salt.
4. Spoon it into 4 bowls, top with the cashews.
5. Serve warm or cold.

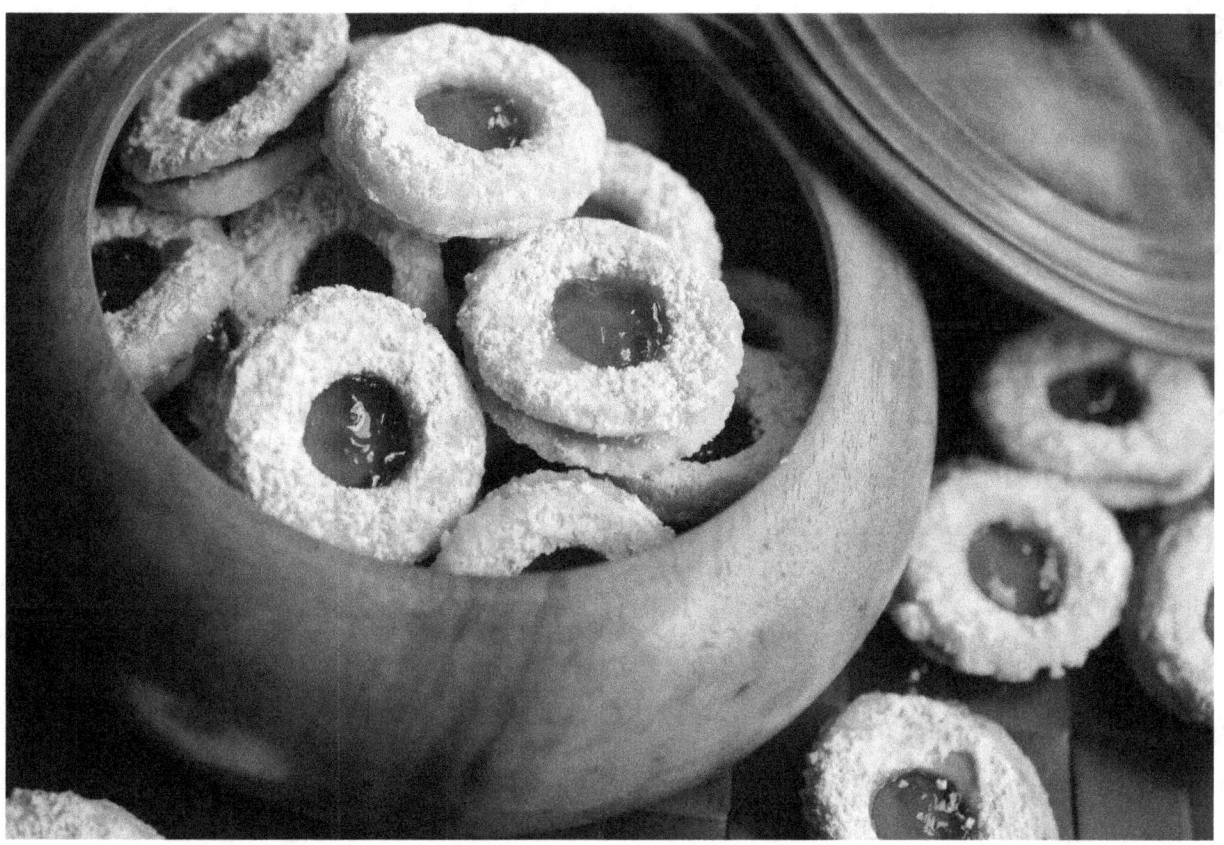

# Pina Colada Cookies

Makes 12-18 cookies

These cookies are a seasonal variation of the Christmas thumbprint cookies. If you do not tolerate pineapple jam, try substituting apricot jam.

**Ingredients**:

1 cup unsalted butter (a dairy free spread will also work)
2/3 cup sugar
1 tsp. vanilla extract
1 tsp. salt

2 cups flour (gluten free flour works also)
1 egg beaten with 1 Tbs. water for egg wash
1 ½ cups sweetened shredded coconut flakes
1 1/3 cups pineapple jam

**Directions**:

1. Beat the butter and sugar together until light and fluffy.
2. Beat in the vanilla, salt, and flour until smooth dough forms.
3. Wrap the dough in plastic wrap and let chill in the refrigerator for 30 minutes.
4. Roll the dough into 1-inch balls.
5. Roll each ball in egg wash and then the coconut flakes.
6. Use your thumb to make an indent in each cookie.
7. Fill each indent with jam.
8. Bake the cookies for 12-15 minutes or until slightly browned.

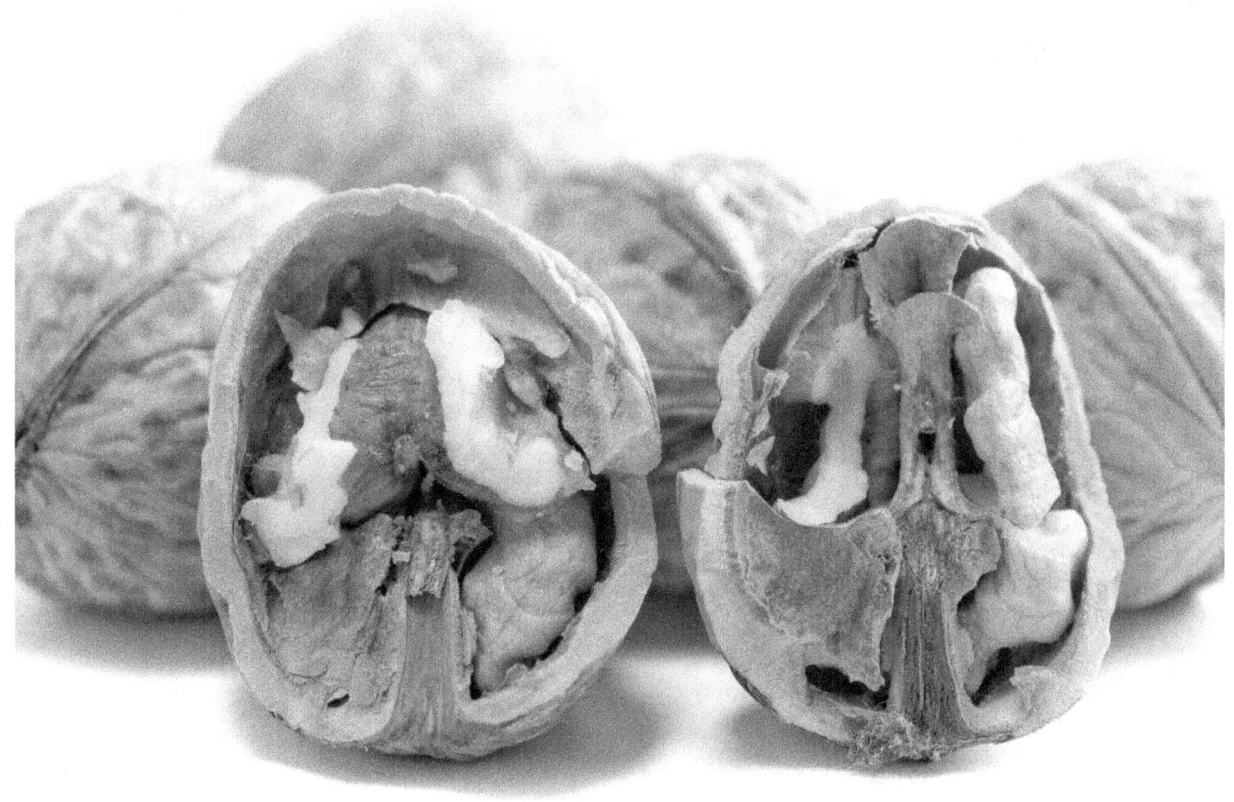

## Walnut Dainties

Makes 3 dozen

Sometimes the simplest recipes are the best for acid reflux disease. Recipes do not get much simpler than this.

**Ingredients**:

2 eggs
2 cups packed brown sugar
2 tsp. vanilla extract
1 cup all-purpose flour

½ tsp baking soda
½ tsp salt
1 cup chopped walnuts

**Directions**:

1. In a bowl, beat the eggs, brown sugar, and vanilla.
2. Combine the flour, baking soda, and salt; add to the egg mixture.
3. Stir in the walnuts.
4. Pour into a greased 13 x 9 inch baking pan.
5. Bake at 350 degrees for 20-25 minutes or until bars pull away from the edges of the pan.

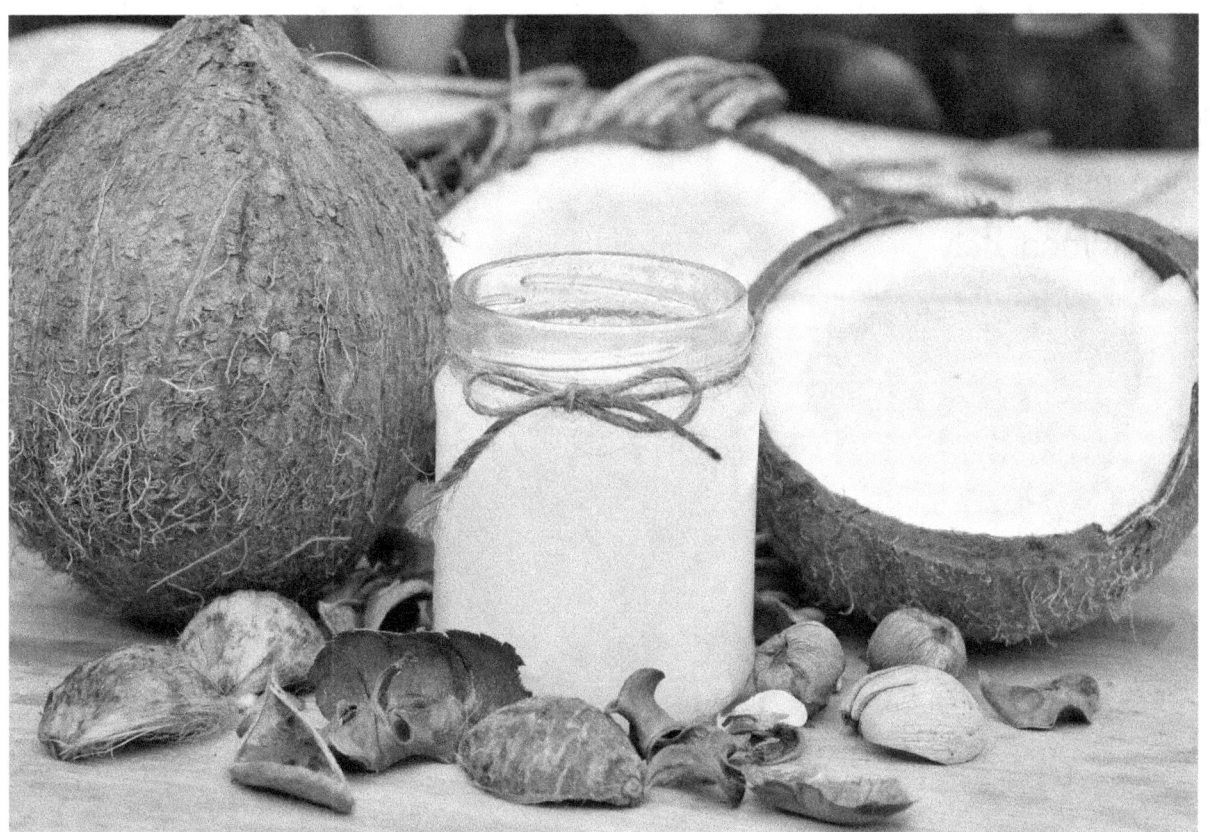

## Coconut Banana Freeze

Serves 4

Bananas have always been a comforting food. The combination of coconut and banana will transport you to the tropics.

**Ingredients**:

5 ripe bananas, sliced and frozen ahead of time
1 15 ounce can coconut milk

**Directions**:

1. Place milk and bananas in a food processor or blender.
2. Blend until smooth.
3. Scoop into four glass bowls.
4. Serve immediately.

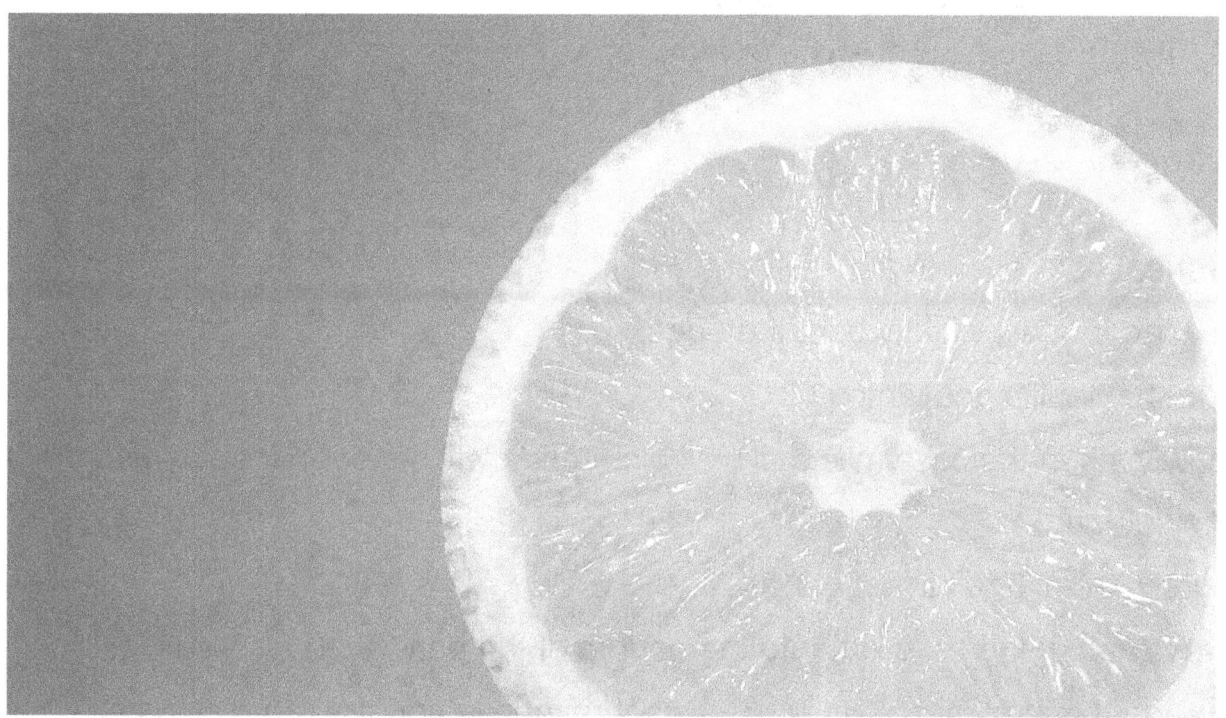

# Jam-Packed Lemon Cake

Makes 1 loaf pan

This was always my go-to cake when my son's reflux was at its worst. He always told me it was the best cake he ever had. It is gluten free, dairy free, and you can use whatever fruit preserves or jam you tolerate the best.

**Ingredients**:

1 package Glutino Old Fashioned Yellow Cake Mix (any brand cake mix will work but I use this mix often in my baking)
½ cup canola oil
2 large eggs

1 tsp. vanilla
1 tsp. lemon oil (or fresh lemon zest)
3 Tbs. of your favorite preserves or jam

**Directions**:

1. Preheat your oven to 350 degrees.
2. In a large bowl, slightly beat the eggs.
3. Add the vanilla and lemon oil.
4. Slowly stir in the cake mix until well blended (it will be a very heavy mix, more like cookie dough).
5. Lightly spray or oil a loaf pan.
6. Press half of the cake mix into the bottom of the pan.
7. Spread the jam on top. Using your fingers, gently add the remaining cake mix on top of the jam.
8. Press the cake mix around to cover the jam (it doesn't have to be perfect).
9. Bake for 20-25 minutes (my son likes it gooey in the middle so you may need to adjust the time based on your preference).

# From Tracy

I wrote this cookbook as a resource for people who have been diagnosed with acid reflux. While different foods can be reflux triggers for different people, there are some foods that are recommended that you avoid with acid reflux. This book should not be used to diagnose yourself or others, rather it will hopefully save you time after your (or your family member's) diagnosis by a health care professional. My hope is that this cookbook will serve as a starting place and will help you feel like you can handle what is now in front of you.

My academic background is in Human Growth and Development, where I earned a Ph.D. focusing on integrated healthcare and disabilities. Maybe even more importantly, I am a parent of a son with acid reflux disease. This book is a compilation of the recipes that I turned to when my son's reflux was at its worst, while at the same time I had another child and a husband to feed. The information contained in this book came from the trenches.

If you have any questions, please do not hesitate to visit my website at TracysHealthyLiving.com. Good luck.

You got this.

www.ingramcontent.com/pod-product-compliance
Lightning Source LLC
Chambersburg PA
CBHW081014170526
45158CB00010B/3031